Allen Carr

The easy way to
lose
weight

ARCTURUS

To Joyce and a squirrel

Editor: Robin Hayley

Additional editorial contributions: Tim Glynne-Jones

ARCTURUS

This edition published in 2016 by Arcturus Publishing Limited
26/27 Bickels Yard, 151–153 Bermondsey Street,
London SE1 3HA, UK

ISBN: 978-1-78404-495-4
AD001650US

Printed in the USA

The easy way to
lose
weight

ALLEN CARR'S EASYWAY

Allen Carr was a chain-smoker for over 30 years. In 1983, after countless failed attempts to quit, he went from 100 cigarettes a day to zero without suffering withdrawal pangs, without using willpower, and without putting on weight. He realized that he had discovered what the world had been waiting for—the Easy Way to Stop Smoking, and embarked on a mission to help cure the world's smokers.

As a result of the phenomenal success of his method, he gained an international reputation as the world's leading expert on stopping smoking and his network of clinics now spans the globe. His first book, *Allen Carr's Easy Way to Stop Smoking*, has sold over 12 million copies, remains an international bestseller and has been published in over 40 different languages. Hundreds of thousands of smokers have successfully quit at Allen Carr's Easyway Clinics where, with a success rate of over 90 percent, he guarantees you'll find it easy to stop or your money back.

Allen Carr's Easyway method has been successfully applied to a host of issues including weight control, alcohol and other drug addictions, worrying, children smoking, and fear of flying.

Weight control, alcohol, and other drug consultations are available at some of Allen Carr's clinics and there is also a full corporate service to help employees and increase productivity in the workplace.

A list of these clinics appears at the back of this book. Should you require any assistance or if you have any questions, please do not hesitate to contact your nearest clinic.

For more information about Allen Carr's Easyway, please visit **www.allencarr.com**

Allen Carr's Easyway

The key that will set you free

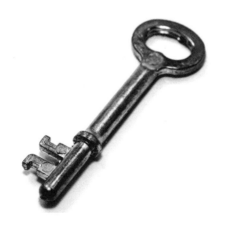

CONTENTS

INTRODUCTION

What I remember most about my early years at school was being teased mercilessly in the playground because I was fat. By the age of 13 the situation had gotten so out of hand that my father took me to Weight Watchers®. I followed the strict regime: weighing everything I ate; using low-calorie powdered milk in my low-calorie cereal; carefully insuring that I didn't exceed the meager rations of butter, cheese, and other high-calorie luxuries allowed. I was surprised at how easy it was to get used to the new foods I was forcing myself to eat. Even the powdered milk, which initially tasted truly awful, soon became perfectly palatable. And I lost weight. However, after the initial novelty had worn off, the whole process began to get me down. Each morning I would wake up thinking about what I was going to allow myself to eat that day. I felt a slave to the diet and found my reserves of willpower gradually being depleted as the lure of forbidden foods increased. And as I lost weight, my motivation to keep to the diet weakened. I felt I deserved to reward myself with the odd chocolate bar or cheese sandwich between meals and so the weight crept back up.

From that time until the age of 35, I fought a continuous battle against weight gain, trying all sorts of diets. Willpower didn't help: for over 20 years my weight went up and down depending on whether I was following a diet or indulging myself. I was so unhappy with my body and so miserable that I was unable to solve the problem that it eventually affected me psychologically and I suffered from various eating disorders. That all changed after I became involved with Allen Carr's Easyway.

In 1989 I had the truly extraordinary experience of stopping smoking easily, painlessly, and permanently at Allen Carr's clinic. I realized at once that Allen Carr had devised a method that could help millions of people all over the world and wrote to him asking to join him in his mission. I was extremely fortunate to be accepted and even luckier later to be appointed Managing Director of the company formed to spread the method all over the world. Today more than 400,000 people have attended our clinics in over 45 countries and Allen Carr's Easyway books have been translated into over 40 languages, have sold more than 16 million copies, and have been read by an estimated 30–40 million people. This phenomenal success has been achieved not through advertising or marketing but through the personal recommendations of the millions of people who have succeeded with the method. Allen Carr's Easyway has spread all over the world for one reason alone: BECAUSE IT WORKS.

Although I didn't put on weight after I stopped smoking with Allen Carr's Easyway, I remained trapped in the continuous struggle to keep it down until Allen applied his method to weight control. Allen and I worked closely together and he asked me for my comments on his first draft of *Allen Carr's Easyweigh To Lose Weight*. I had no idea it was going to transform my life so radically for the better. As I read through the text, I found the powerful logic irrefutable. By the end I knew that my weight problem was solved. No longer did I have to use willpower to deny myself forbidden foods. No longer did I have to weigh what I ate. No longer did I have to feel deprived because I couldn't eat as much as I wanted or guilty because I had eaten too much. Gone was the tug-of-war in my mind that made the whole issue of food and eating such a nightmare. By following Allen's instructions, I escaped from that slavery and found it easy to reach and stay at my ideal weight. Far from feeling miserable or deprived, I enjoyed the process right from the start. It was a revelation to me that I didn't have to avoid food to be thin and that I could look forward to and enjoy eating, and still be my ideal weight.

Waking up in the morning full of energy and free to eat whatever you like is such a liberating experience! Seeing your slim body in the mirror and knowing that you never have to worry about it expanding again is truly wonderful! That's the marvelous transformation that happened to me.

The Easy Way to Lose Weight presents Allen Carr's method in a new, updated, and easily accessible format, which, with the added help of a hypnotherapy CD, makes it even simpler and more enjoyable to solve your weight problem. I very much hope it transforms your life in the fantastic way it has transformed mine.

Robin Hayley M.A. (Oxon), M.B.A., M.A.A.C.T.I.
Managing Director, Allen Carr's Easyway (International) Ltd

CHAPTER 1

THE KEY

IN THIS CHAPTER

• THIS BOOK IS THE KEY TO SOLVING YOUR WEIGHT PROBLEM
• JUNK FOOD • THE SMOKING CONNECTION • WILLPOWER
• THE FIRST INSTRUCTION

Eat as much of your favorite foods as you want, whenever you want, as often as you want, and be the exact weight you want to be without dieting, special exercise, using willpower, or feeling deprived

Do you find it hard to imagine that could possibly be achievable? I promise you it is. By reading this book with an open mind you will discover a wonderful new life that may now seem beyond your dreams: a life in which you enjoy every meal, in which you are slim, fit, healthy, and bursting with an energy you had forgotten even existed; an active, sociable, long, and happy life. And achieving that new life will be easy.

Maybe you think that's too good to be true. Perhaps it goes against everything you've ever been told about weight loss. Has what you've been told before worked for you? If it had, you wouldn't be reading this book.

Eating is one of life's great pleasures. We look forward to

mealtimes with excitement; we shop for food with anticipation; we celebrate our achievements, tout for business, and court prospective lovers by booking a table at a restaurant, or preparing something special at home. Few human customs have survived the test of time quite like the feast. For thousands of years we have associated food and eating with good times.

Yet how often do you feel good after a meal? I always thought of myself as a food lover. I was the ideal dinner guest—a big eater who wasn't fussy. And yet more often than not, when I finished a meal it wasn't with a feeling of joy or satisfaction but one of both physical and mental discomfort.

I didn't really taste what I ate. I just shoveled it down. My belly would feel bloated and tight like a drum. I frequently suffered from indigestion and heartburn, and even worse was my guilt and helplessness as I loosened a button or two while cursing myself for ending up in this condition yet again.

You'd think that would be enough to put anyone off overeating for a while. Yet by the time the next mealtime came around, I'd be back to square one and going through the same torture all over again.

I knew I ate too much, I only had to look at my ever-expanding belly in the mirror to see that. I had never regarded eating and overeating as separate entities. To me overeating was merely an extension of eating, probably caused by the fact that I liked eating so much. Smokers believe the problems they have quitting are because they enjoy smoking so much. In fact they never do. They only believe they do because they feel miserable and deprived when they're not allowed to smoke. In the same way, overeaters believe their problem is that they enjoy eating too much. You might well feel miserable and deprived whenever you're not allowed to eat as much as you want, but that doesn't mean you enjoy overeating.

As you probably know, I'm famous for discovering a method that enables any smoker to find it easy and enjoyable to quit. I was a smoker for 33 years. I tried to quit many times by using willpower but always fell back into the trap. I was convinced that I couldn't cope with or enjoy life without smoking, but I longed to be free. When I finally quit permanently, it took no willpower, I didn't feel deprived, and I never missed it. Today I'm widely accepted as the world's leading stop-smoking expert. My book *Allen Carr's Easy Way to Stop Smoking* has sold over 12 million copies and we have a worldwide clinic network.

I learned about the nature of addiction by quitting smoking. What I wasn't aware of was that I was also addicted to the processed sugar in junk food, and that was one of the major causes of my overeating. It was the simple realization that smoking was an addiction, not something I did for pleasure, that enabled me to discover my stop-smoking method and escape from that prison. I later realized that the method also works for other addictions and problems, including overeating.

MAKING THE CONNECTION

I must admit I didn't see it that way to begin with. While I could see quite clearly that my method could be applied to alcohol and all drug addictions, applying it to food initially stretched my mind. There were two reasons for this. First, at the heart of the method is the fact that it's easy to quit smoking completely, but it requires incredible willpower to cut down or control your intake. Obviously cutting out food completely is out of the question! Second, I knew that eating can be a genuine pleasure and does actually satisfy hunger, whereas the pleasure of smoking is an illusion and the cigarette creates the hunger it seems to relieve.

But through my discovery of the way to escape the smoking trap, I realized that I had been the victim of brainwashing from the day I was born and that applied to eating as much as it did to smoking.

> **••• FACT BOX •••**
> In 2014, the World Health Organization estimated that 1.9 billion adults were overweight, and it predicted this figure would rise. In the developed world over 50% of adults are overweight. In the U.S.A., the figure is over 70%. The percentage of overweight children in the developed world has more than doubled in the last 40 years, from around 10% to over 20% today.
> This is a modern problem, coinciding with the boom in junk foods over the last 50 years.

The tobacco industry is hugely powerful and feeds us lies and illusions in ingeniously subtle ways. Just as powerful as Big Tobacco is the food industry. If Big Food simply produced the food we need to keep fit and healthy, it wouldn't be anything like the size it is, nor would we! The fact is that the food industry encourages us to overeat.

If the supermarket only stocked the natural foods that we genuinely enjoy and need to be healthy, fit, and happy, its fat profits would shrink. The vast bulk of food on supermarket shelves is surplus to our requirements. When I felt that my method could not be applied to weight loss, I was overlooking a crucial point. I was comparing smoking to eating: the first a disgusting, smelly, unhealthy, antisocial addiction that makes us feel terrible and gives us no benefits whatsoever; the second an enjoyable, sociable activity that satisfies our hunger, gives us energy, and keeps us alive.

EUREKA

What I should have been comparing it to was not eating but overeating. It was like a lightbulb coming on in my brain—a Eureka moment, just like the time I decided to embark on my mission to cure the world of smoking. Until I saw the light, I had regarded overeating as a mere extension of eating: too much of a good thing. I now realized that the two were entirely different.

The effects of overeating have a lot in common with the effects of smoking. On the physical side: tiredness and lethargy; indigestion and heartburn; lack of fitness; obesity; heart disease; and all sorts of other life-threatening illnesses. On the mental side: an illusion of pleasure; guilt; helplessness; lack of self-esteem and sex drive; slavery and misery.

So I asked myself the question: Since smoking is caused by an addiction to nicotine, is overeating caused by eating junk food and an addiction to processed sugar? And the more I thought about it, the more I realized this was the case.

The yo-yo effect

Diets restrict your intake of food in an attempt to help you lose weight. Usually people who fall into the trap of trying to solve their weight problem by dieting end up in a vicious circle known as "the yo-yo effect": an endless cycle of restricting your intake to lose weight, putting on weight again once you start to eat more, and then restricting your intake again to lose the weight once more. It's very unhealthy for your body to expand and shrink over and over again. Worse, your life is dominated by having constantly to think about what, when, and how much you can allow yourself to eat. Dieting is a nightmare and will never solve your weight problem.

With my method you will not have to change your lifestyle. You will be able to go out to eat with friends and family and enjoy other social events without feeling deprived.

I mentioned before that it's much harder to cut down than to quit because cutting down requires willpower. And not just a bit of willpower for a few days or weeks, it requires an immense amount of willpower for the rest of your life.

On the other hand, quitting altogether requires no willpower at all provided you don't feel you're making a sacrifice. In fact, it's easy. This applies to overeating. All you have to do is reverse the brainwashing that has led you to believe that overeating is pleasurable. If you try to cut down, you perpetuate the illusion that you're being deprived and you become miserable and irritable. Junk food becomes more and more precious and you become convinced that the only way to feel better is to stuff your face. Eventually you reach breaking point. You tell yourself that you deserve a reward and go on a binge, undoing all the hard work you put in. It's the same story with every diet:

DIETS DON'T WORK

My method for losing weight is not a diet. When I use the term "diet" in this book, I am referring to the restrictive regime we go on to lose weight through willpower. "Diet" can also mean the total food that one consumes, i.e. your intake. However, to avoid confusion, I will refer to that as "intake."

The problem is not eating but overeating. This may give you the impression that the issue is simply the amount you consume and that you need to eat less. No, the problem is not so much the quantity of food you eat as the type. Perhaps you fear that you will no longer be allowed to eat your favorite foods. Not so. If you follow the simple guidelines in this book, you will be able to eat as much of your favorite foods as you want without being overweight. What's more, you will not need to count calories, weigh your food, or limit your intake by using willpower.

So why don't I just give you the instructions now? I wish I could. I want to help you as quickly as possible, but in order to be happy to follow the instructions, you first need to understand the method. There's no need to worry; this won't take long and you'll enjoy the journey.

As we go through this book, I will give you the simple instructions that will set you free. It's essential that you follow them and understand them. And that's the first instruction:

FOLLOW ALL THE INSTRUCTIONS

If there's anything you don't understand, go back and read it again until it becomes clear. I want you to get the maximum pleasure and enjoyment out of life, not to make you suffer or feel deprived. So carry on eating as you normally do while you read this book and by the end you'll have the joy of knowing that your weight problem is solved.

SUMMARY

- My method is easy.
- Eating is a pleasure.
- Overeating is a pain.
- Dieting will not solve the problem, it will only make it worse.
- Follow all the instructions and you will find the key.

TOP TIP No.1

The Pleasure of Eating

Eating is one of life's great pleasures. If you eat natural foods, which are easy to digest, your body will work efficiently and you will be your correct weight. You will neither feel bloated nor have indigestion. Real food is eaten in its natural state. Junk is processed, often with chemicals and unnatural additives and preservatives. Follow my method and you will learn to recognize the difference between food and junk. You will enjoy maximum pleasure from eating, become slim, and stay that way.

CHAPTER 2

IN A NUTSHELL

IN THIS CHAPTER
- *THE SQUIRREL*
- *WILD ANIMALS ARE NOT OVERWEIGHT*
- *THE SECOND INSTRUCTION*

LEARNING FROM NATURE

It's funny how the most everyday occurrences can trigger the most important discoveries. Isaac Newton had his moment of inspiration when an apple fell from a tree. For me, it was a squirrel that provided the crucial piece of evidence that enabled me to discover the secret of weight control

There was nothing unusual about a squirrel coming into my garden. We had daily visits, encouraged by the peanuts that my wife Joyce would generously scatter on the patio. We always enjoyed watching it performing fantastic acrobatics, its agility being a constant source of wonder. Our cat was fascinated too, albeit for different reasons.

I find it difficult to love my cat when she's hunting some small, hapless animal. It's bad enough when it's one of those strident starlings, but when it's a robin or a blue tit I find it impossible. On one occasion I watched as she crept up and cornered a squirrel

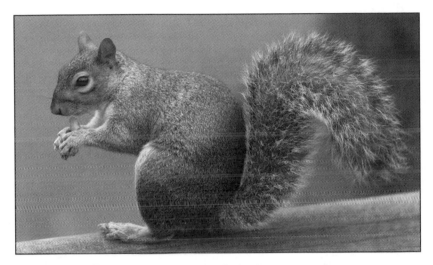

The squirrel knows instinctively when to stop eating

against the wall of the neighbor's house. I couldn't see any way out for the squirrel without a fight, and watched with interest to see how the cat would fare against this tough and nimble opponent. The squirrel simply turned and ran up the vertical wall.

A few days later I looked out of the window and saw the squirrel sitting on the patio, happily eating the nuts that Joyce had put out. My mind went back to the incident with the cat and I thought to myself, "Eat too many of those and there's no way you'll be able to climb the wall next time!" As if it had read my mind, the squirrel immediately stopped eating the nuts and started burying them.

I couldn't stop wondering why the squirrel had chosen to stop eating and start storing. If Joyce had put a bowl of peanuts in front of me, I would have scoffed all of them. I was aware that gorging myself on snacks wasn't doing my figure any favors—so what?

I wasn't planning to rush up any vertical walls in the foreseeable future.

But there was something I couldn't understand: If I couldn't stop eating, how could the squirrel? Here was I, a member of the most intelligent species on the planet, being outsmarted by a mere rodent.

For several days I found myself pondering what I had witnessed in the garden. I had no problem understanding the squirrel's behavior. Anyone could see the sense in keeping some food back for later if you're a creature that can never be sure where your next meal is coming from. But how could the squirrel see that? How could an animal with a brain not much bigger than the nuts it was eating have the foresight to stop eating when food was abundant and store it away for later? Did it know that if it overate it wouldn't be able to scale the wall to escape the cat in future? Was that why it didn't have a weight problem?

The picture started to become clearer in my mind when I realized that not only had I never seen a squirrel with a weight problem, I had never seen a wild animal of any species that was overweight. Sure, there are animals like walruses and hippos that seem fat, but that's the shape that Nature intended. It suits their lifestyle and the environment in which they live. I have never seen a walrus or hippo that is distinctly overweight compared to the rest of the herd.

Think of the amazing images we see of animals in large groups. It could be a school of fish, a herd of water buffalo, a flock of geese. Their individual sizes may differ, but they're all the same shape, the same proportion. There are none that lag behind the others, weighed down by an oversized belly caused by overeating.

•••• **FACT BOX** ••••

50% of humans in the developed world are overweight

0% of wild animals are overweight

It dawned on me that human intelligence isn't the only thing that sets us apart from the animal kingdom. We are also the only species on the planet that has weight problems; we and the domesticated animals whose eating habits we control.

This was my "Eureka!" moment. It was an overwhelming piece of evidence: 99.99% of all creatures on Earth eat as much of their favorite foods as they want, as often as they want, without being overweight. Obviously there was a simple secret, simple enough for a squirrel to comprehend and yet the most intelligent species on the planet hadn't worked it out.

Could it be that, by some ironic twist, intelligence has become the very reason for our ignorance? Perhaps the fact that we have more brainpower than any other species has led us away from the truth. There's no shortage of fables that warn how arrogance and complacency can lead us to overlook the simplest truths.

Why do we need nutritionists to tell us what to eat to keep in shape? Animals don't, they know instinctively what they should and shouldn't eat. And so did we once upon a time. Our intellect has led us to think differently, so differently that it has overridden the wisdom of our instincts.

FOLLOW YOUR INSTINCTS

There are so many contradictory diet books, no wonder we're confused. They're full of technical information and statistics that even scientists can't fully understand. In fact, all that technical detail is an effort to blind us to the inadequacies of the diets themselves. The only information we really need is the information we were born with: instinct.

It wasn't intelligence that made the squirrel stop eating, it was instinct. And it was observing the squirrel that made me think how nice it would be to be able to eat as much of your favorite foods as you want, whenever you want, as often as you want, and be the exact weight you want to be without dieting, special exercise, using willpower, or feeling deprived.

When I first presented you with this idea, you may have thought it sounded too good to be true. When is life ever that simple? In fact, 99.99% of the animal kingdom finds it that simple. Let's take a closer look and discover how they do it.

You might point to the difficulty animals have in finding food and taking it back to their families. Yes, food is often scarce and that can restrict their consumption and even lead to starvation. But what about when food is abundant? Why don't you see animals gorging themselves and getting fat? I've already told you about the squirrel. Another good example is the termite.

Termites feast on rotten wood. That may not strike you as a mouthwatering choice, and you could argue that you wouldn't be overweight either if that was all you ate! To the termite rotten wood is the nectar of the gods. It's their favorite food and there's no shortage of it. Yet termites do not get overweight. They don't keep eating until they can no longer move. Somehow they know when to stop.

Before we look more closely at the reasons why humans have departed from the rest of the animal kingdom in this respect, I want to point out that Allen Carr's Easyway method isn't magic. Like those who have quit smoking, some people who have lost weight by this method have described it as such, but that's purely a figure of speech. There's nothing mysterious about my method. It's not magic and it's not a diet. I will not be asking you to control your intake by using willpower. By reading this book you will understand that overeating is a consequence of incorrect eating.

I'm not asking you simply to trust me or have faith. I am asking you to keep an open mind. Provided you understand the fundamental principles of the method, you will also understand the reasons behind my instructions and then you will find it easy and enjoyable to follow them. The second instruction is:

KEEP AN OPEN MIND

This is very important. I have yet to meet a person who will admit to having a closed mind. You may be convinced that you have an open mind, in which case the chances are it's closed. If you're already convinced, you're not open to other possibilities. By taking a relaxed approach and using your common sense, you will open your mind, your fears will dissolve, and you will find it easy to understand and follow my method.

Are you seeing straight?

Look at the figure below. What do you see?

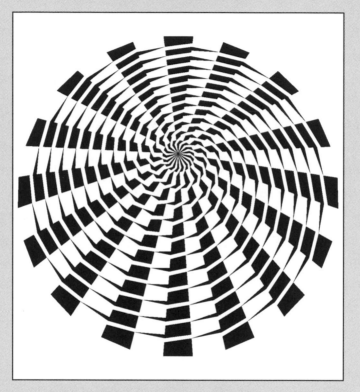

If you think you see a spiral, look again. In fact, it's a series of concentric circles. Your eyes are picking up characteristics that you associate with a spiral and your brain is jumping to the conclusion that it is a spiral. It shows how quick we are to fall back on what we have learned to be true, rather than looking at each new picture with fresh eyes and an open mind.

In order to open your mind, first you need to realize it has been closed.

I always thought of myself as open-minded. When I discovered the secret to being slim, fit, and healthy, I couldn't understand how I had closed my mind to such obvious facts for so many years. It was an enormous relief to open my mind and free myself from my weight problem.

SUMMARY

- Animals stop eating when their hunger is satisfied.
- The only species that have weight problems are humans and their domesticated animals.
- Our intellect overrides the wisdom of our instincts.
- The secret to correct eating is simple: 99.99% of animals understand it.
- Easyway is not a diet.
- Open your mind by accepting that it may have been closed.

Top Tip No.2

Follow your Instincts

99.99% of animals eat as much of their favorite foods as they want, as often as they, want without being overweight. Learn which foods best suit you. You will not solve your weight problem by dieting, which requires willpower and makes you feel deprived.

CHAPTER 3

THE BRAINWASHING

IN THIS CHAPTER
• *DO YOU CHOOSE WHAT YOU EAT?*
• *WHY DIETS DON'T WORK*
• *THE THIRD INSTRUCTION*

EMPOWER NOT WILLPOWER

You have not chosen the way you eat now, it's the result of a lifetime's brainwashing

Although I thought of myself as a food lover, I wasn't happy with my eating habits. The anticipation I felt before a meal was not matched by a feeling of satisfaction afterward. I knew there was something wrong, but I couldn't seem to change the way I ate and it made me feel stupid and inadequate.

I now know there was nothing to be ashamed of. Overeaters are not being foolish, because the "choices" they make when it comes to eating are not free choices at all. They're the result of a lifetime's brainwashing. The vast majority of meals you've consumed since the day you were born were not chosen by you. Since you haven't been the one in charge, there's no reason for you to feel responsible for the way your eating habits have evolved.

Now you're going to take charge of what you eat. You know

there's something wrong with your eating habits, but you don't know how to change them. The first thing to get clear in your mind is that you're changing a situation that you're unhappy with for the purely selfish reason that you'll enjoy life infinitely more.

People usually feel a sense of doom and gloom whenever they try to solve their weight problem because they believe it means going on a diet, or doing a course of strenuous exercise, or both. It's a daunting and miserable prospect, requiring massive willpower.

Fortunately there's a simple and enjoyable alternative: Allen Carr's Easyway. It requires no willpower, nor does it restrict you to eating food you don't enjoy, nor require you to follow an exercise program. All you have to do is understand and follow the method and you'll find yourself automatically changing your eating habits and enjoying the process.

Many of you will have tried to lose weight by going on a diet. If you've been a keen follower of a low-calorie weight loss regime the chances are that you're undernourished, your digestion is poor, and your health below par. With my method you'll be eating what you want and getting all the nourishment you need. Your digestion will be working at its optimum and you will lose weight.

THE TASTE OF FREEDOM

Perhaps you think I'm moving the goalposts by saying that you'll be changing the way you eat. If you think you already eat as much of your favorite foods as you want, and that's why you have a weight problem in the first place, think again. Remember the optical illusion in the previous chapter. What you thought was a spiral was actually a series of concentric circles. Let's look at your favorite foods with an open mind.

The foods you currently consider to be your favorites aren't making you happy. If they were, you wouldn't be reading this book. What kind of favorite is it that makes you unhappy? Remember, your eating habits have been controlled by others from the day you were born. It's time to make your own choices.

If you think the foods you currrently consider to be your favorites are the foods that taste the best, open your mind. The beautiful truth is that the foods that taste best are, in fact, the best for you. You find this hard to believe because you've been brainwashed by the junk food manufacturers.

Taste is easily led astray. Many luxury foods taste revolting initially. Take oysters, for example. Oysters used to be a poor man's staple, and it's not hard to see why. Who in their right mind would eat something with the consistency of phlegm and the flavor of salt water unless they had to? The same applies to caviar, foie gras, and a whole host of expensive delicacies that taste repugnant to anyone trying them for the first time.

Have you ever eaten a hamburger and really focused on the flavors in your mouth? Now, if I told you the burger was made of dog meat, how do you think that would change your perception of the taste? I bet you'd spit it out pretty fast. Why? Is there any logical reason we should regard a cow, which spends its life covered in mud, excrement, and flies, as something tasty to eat, while the thought of eating dog appalls us? If so, why is the perception reversed in other cultures, where cows are sacred and dogs are seen as meat?

Don't worry, I'm not about to claim that eating dog is the answer to your weight problem! I'm merely illustrating how we're brainwashed about what is, and isn't, good to eat. Is it the cow-eaters or the dog-eaters who've been brainwashed? The answer is both. It shows how susceptible we are to conditioning, for better or for worse.

The rat trap

Rats are seen as dirty, disease-ridden, vicious creatures. The hamster, on the other hand, is regarded as a cute, cuddly little ball of fur. Yet the rat and the hamster are both rodents and actually look very similar. People who have pet rats will tell you they're clean, intelligent, and every bit as pleasant to keep as a hamster, which, given half a chance, will give you a nasty nip with its razor-sharp teeth.

We regard some animals as our friends and others as our enemies. We don't realize we've been brainwashed. Dogs inflict twice as many fatal attacks on humans as sharks, yet we regard the dog as man's best friend and the shark as our mortal enemy. When it comes to food, our perceptions are also seldom based on fact and logic; they're more often an emotional response to our conditioning through books, films, TV, advertisements, and popular mythology.

WHY WE EAT JUNK

From birth our eating habits are controlled by others. Think about it: were you breast-fed as a baby or given the bottle? Whose decision was that? Who decided when it was time to wean you off milk and move you on to solids?

As you grew older, did you decide the school menu or the contents of your lunchbox? At work, can you choose anything you like for lunch? And even when you come home, do you decide what you're having for dinner? Even if you're doing the cooking, you're still restricted by your budget and what's available.

Most of the meals we've eaten since the day we were born were not the result of our personal choice. We eat according to the influences of our upbringing.

You might be thinking, "My problem isn't the meals I eat, it's the snacking in-between, the candy I pick up at the check-out. Surely that's my own free will?"

It isn't. Your desire to pick up a chocolate bar is triggered by an association in your mind created by advertising. The junk food marketeers are only interested in selling as much of their addictive poisons to as many people as possible. There's no limit to the claims they'll make, often in fiendishly subtle ways, to create the impression that this lethal combination of sugar and fat gives you energy, heightened sex appeal, and makes you cool. Some are even sold at certain times of year only, such as limited-edition summer ice cream flavors, as if they're a seasonal product like fruit! They aren't interested in your figure, health, well-being or happiness, only in getting you hooked.

Once the false image is planted in your mind, any association can trigger the desire for junk. You might hear the jingle from a chocolate bar ad or see a car pass by featured in an ice cream commercial.

THIS ISN'T CHOICE, IT'S BRAINWASHING

We're often not even in control of the amount we eat. If you're anything like I was, you'll polish off everything on your plate. We're conditioned to think it's rude or picky to leave food that somebody else has prepared for us. Do you decide how much is put on the plate? When you're serving, do you know how hungry others are or what they want to eat? Do you pile the food up high so as not to appear stingy?

All over the world, celebrations are marked by eating too much. Christmas lunch is a prime example. Even people who normally eat a moderate amount suddenly find themselves with a plate piled high with turkey, stuffing and several different vegetables, all drowned in gravy, and cranberry sauce.

And as if that weren't enough, they then have to find room for a special, usually very rich, dessert. And they feel compelled to consume it all. On a day when you should be having a wonderful time with your family, you end up bloated and lethargic, full of food which is supposed to give you pleasure but in reality does the opposite. Your kidneys and liver can't remove all the toxins and your stomach, intestines, and bowels can't cope with the overload. This toxic surplus has to be stored in your body as fat.

From now on you're going to be the one in control of what you eat, rather than the other way around. You will decide what your favorite foods are. You will decide how much you consume and how often. You will be able to:

Eat as much of your favorite foods as you want, whenever you want, as often as you want, and be the exact weight you want to be, without dieting, special exercise, using willpower, or feeling deprived

When most people read this they assume there must be a catch. I assure you there isn't. If it were too good to be true, 99.99% of creatures on this planet wouldn't be doing it. If it works for them, surely it can work for you. What do you have to lose by trying? Can you honestly say that you enjoy every meal you eat now? Take a moment to look at all the benefits I'm offering. In addition to the added pleasure you'll enjoy from eating, you'll feel lighter, healthier, more energetic and self-confident, and you will never again suffer that horrible guilty feeling.

What's more, because this isn't a diet, you won't have to go through the soul-destroying process of counting calories. When you think about the miserable business of measuring out your meagre, daily allowance of butter or sugar, it's no wonder that it ends in failure. The basic flaw with diets is they're short term. My method is designed to remove your problem permanently without willpower or feeling deprived. If you know people who seem to control their weight by dieting, don't be fooled into thinking they've succeeded in solving their problem. The fact that they have to resist the temptation of the donut makes it far more precious to them, and when they eventually run out of willpower, they balloon in size.

If I asked you to stand on one leg with the other leg held up behind you, you'd probably think that's easy. What if I then asked you to hold your other leg up too without falling over? You'd think I was being ridiculous. You wouldn't consider yourself a failure for not being able to do it. It's impossible.

As long as you feel you're making a sacrifice, you will never become free. Don't worry, with my method, you will solve your weight problem without feeling deprived or miserable and you will be free to enjoy life to the full.

When you go on a diet, you're being asked to do the impossible. This isn't obvious, because to begin with you can achieve some success, which suggests the diet works. In fact it only works as long as your willpower lasts.

When you restrict your eating, you feel permanently hungry. You become obsessed with the thought of your next meal, and when it comes it's a huge anticlimax. Compared to what you were used to eating, it's neither exciting, nor enough, and you're left feeling miserable again. Dissatisfied, you eat slightly more than the diet allows, which makes you feel guilty.

It has been established that most people who attempt to lose weight through dieting actually gain weight in the long term. Diets make food appear more precious. And if you finally reach your target weight, what are you meant to do then? Do you go on with the diet? Of course not. You're happy with the weight you are and there's no way you're going to keep to the miserable rations it put you on. So you abandon the diet and go back to your old eating habits. In a fraction of the time it took you to lose the weight, you've put it all back on and more.

It's virtually impossible to lose weight permanently by dieting and the process itself is a nightmare. Your failures in the past were not caused by any deficiency on your part but simply because you were using the wrong method.

Remember, the purpose of my method is to enable you to get maximum enjoyment out of life. The way you've been eating up until now has made you miserable. We're going to help you change that for good. This is cause for celebration. Keep a positive attitude at all times. All you have to do is follow my method. The third instruction is:

START OFF WITH A FEELING OF EXCITEMENT

Forget about the past, look forward to the future, and cast off any sense of doom or gloom. Nothing bad is happening. On the contrary, something marvelous is taking place. You are about to reverse a lifetime's brainwashing, attain your ideal weight, and start enjoying life to the full.

SUMMARY

- The way you eat now is a source of misery, not happiness.
- You've been brainwashed into thinking junk is your favorite food.
- Big Food isn't interested in your wellbeing.
- Let's reverse the brainwashing.
- Something exciting is happening in your life.

Top Tip No.3

Beware of any Food that has an Ingredients List

Food with an ingredients list is processed. Over 17,000 new products appear on the supermarket shelves each year. Big Food achieves this range by subtly changing the ingredients list on the package. Don't be fooled, it's all junk.

CHAPTER 4

THE INCREDIBLE MACHINE

IN THIS CHAPTER
• *THE HUMAN BODY AND THE CAR* • *NATURE'S GUIDE*
• *WHERE HAS OUR INTELLIGENCE GOTTEN US?*
• *THE FOURTH INSTRUCTION*

FOOD FOR THOUGHT

Our body is infinitely more complex than any machine made by humans,
and yet we assume humans are the experts on how to maintain it

There are two basic comparisons that help to clarify the thinking
behind my method. The first is between humans and wild animals.
Remarkably, 99.99% of the animal kingdom, like the squirrel in
my garden, have the secret to eating their favorite foods whenever
they want while remaining their ideal weight.

The second comparison is between our body and a car. They
have a lot in common. They have similar basic requirements in order
to perform their functions; neither can operate without sufficient
supplies of fuel and air and both need to be maintained correctly.

Don't worry if you don't have a degree in mechanical
engineering or a Ph.D. in medicine, I have no intention of blinding
you with science. Even if you haven't learned to drive, you'll find
this very easy to follow.

The car is a fairly complex piece of machinery, but compared to your body it's about as sophisticated as an old-fashioned typewriter compared to a modern laptop. The sophistication of the modern car is certainly impressive; look after it carefully and it might last you 15 years. Now consider your body. Looked after carefully, how long do you think it might last? Currently, 67 years is the world's average life expectancy for human beings.

Say if I asked you to blink your right eye. No problem. But what if I had to get every one of the seven billion people on the planet to blink their right eye at the same time? Even with the full might of modern communication systems, it's an impossible task. And yet a similar feat takes place continuously inside your body.

Your lungs breathe in air, extract the oxygen, and pass it on to the bloodstream; your heart pumps steadily and consistently to distribute that oxygenated blood to every part of your body; your digestive system breaks down food, sorts the nutrients from the waste matter, and sends them on their way; your immune system fights off infection and repairs injuries; and your internal thermostat makes sure that your body maintains its optimum temperature.

Provided it's working properly, your body carries out these incredibly complex functions automatically, whether you're awake or asleep. Because they happen without any conscious effort on our part, we take it all for granted. Fortunately, we don't all have to understand the finer points of the internal combustion engine. When we buy a car the experts provide a manufacturer's handbook. All we have to do is follow the instructions.

HUMANS DESIGNED THE CAR BUT THEY DIDN'T DESIGN THEMSELVES

Humans have designed many amazing things but they didn't design the most amazing creation on Earth: the human being itself.

Whether you believe it was God who created humans, or that we evolved by natural selection over billions of years, or a combination of the two, it's clear that whoever or whatever force created our minds and bodies was infinitely more sophisticated than we are.

So how did it expect us to know how to keep our bodies running smoothly? Who are we supposed to turn to for instructions? From birth, it's humans who decide what we eat. How do humans know? We are informed by dieticians, doctors, nutritionists, and, more than anything else, from persuasive advertising and brainwashing by the junk food industry. Do you really think these people know best?

Of course they don't, so what alternative do we have? Why, you may wonder, didn't the superior force that designed us in the first place provide us with our own manufacturer's handbook? That way we could know automatically what we should eat and when, without having to try and find the truth hidden amid the mass of contradictory information we're constantly fed by so-called experts.

I have good news for you: it did.

Our creator, who or whatever it was, provided all living creatures with a manufacturer's handbook. I'll refer to it from now on as Nature's Guide. It's how our ancestors survived long before the supermarket, the ready meal, the microwave, and the dietician came on the scene. Our forefathers didn't need to be told about calories and vitamins, any more than you need to be told about the workings of the internal combustion engine for you to keep your car running.

Nature's Guide is what wild animals follow and that's how they effortlessly maintain their ideal weight.

You may feel there's a glaring contradiction in what I'm saying. On one hand I've talked about the superiority of humans, and on the other I appear to be suggesting that we have much to learn from wild animals. That's exactly what I'm saying, but there's no contradiction.

> *Our intellect has enabled us to establish superiority over other animals. Intelligence is a wonderful thing, but it can go to your head. Nature has provided us with a bounty of privileges and opportunities; is there anything wrong with using our intelligence to improve things even further? Not if we really are improving them. Look again at the so-called advances we've made, including in our eating habits, and they show we've gone against Nature's Guide.*

WHERE HAS OUR INTELLIGENCE GOTTEN US?

We use the word "animalistic" to describe human behavior that we believe to be inhuman: mindless violence, vandalism, wanton destruction. And yet this sort of behavior is exclusively human. In fact, we have applied some of the finest minds in history to the quest for destruction, resulting in bombs that could destroy the entire planet.

The atomic bomb was supposed to be the ultimate deterrent to spell the end of war forever. And yet it failed to prevent the carnage in Vietnam or the Balkans, Iraq, Afghanistan, or any of the other numerous conflicts that have broken out since World War II ended.

The idea of destroying the planet with bombs is abhorrent to all of us, and yet we have inflicted untold damage through other means in the name of progress: the pollution and destruction of our natural environment through deforestation, overmining, overfarming, overfishing, and urbanization.

We have made spectacular breakthroughs in medicine, but many of the diseases we treat are the result of ignoring our instinct and thereby Nature.

Is this progress?

THE WRONG FOODS

I suffered from constipation for years. I accepted it as an annoying but common fact of life. Each time I went to my doctor he would prescribe me some medicine and within a few days the constipation would go. But it kept coming back. It never crossed my mind to try to find out why I was getting constipated in the first place. The human body clearly isn't designed to suffer recurring constipation. Why didn't it occur to me that I was eating the wrong foods? Why didn't my doctor tell me?

We've come to accept all manner of ailments as a normal

part of life—indigestion, heartburn, constipation, diarrhoea, headaches, kidney stones, Type 2 diabetes, gout, nausea—we take our medicine and, if we're lucky, the symptoms disappear. Rather than simply treating symptoms, we should look for the root cause. If we have a flat tire, we don't just pump it up and wait for it to go flat again; we do everything possible to find the cause of the puncture and repair it.

If the oil warning light on your car's dashboard comes on, what do you do? Remove the bulb? Of course not! You top up the oil. All the symptoms I've mentioned are warning lights, indications that something is wrong, and to solve the problem we need to address the cause.

Our symptoms are part of Nature's Guide. Treat them with a "magic pill" that prevents your brain from registering them and you are removing the Guide.

Some symptoms, such as vomiting or coughing, are also part of the cure, Nature's method of ejecting poisons from the stomach or lungs. Take a pill to remove those symptoms and you are actively hindering the cure.

Many of the medicines that doctors prescribe actually make matters worse. Painkillers have side effects which cause serious problems. Drugs are poisons administered in controlled doses. The body reacts to the poison, building an immunity to it. As a result, stronger and stronger doses of the drug are required to mask the pain, until it no longer works. The original problem has not been eradicated, the patient is again in pain, and now they're also addicted to the painkillers.

Blinded by science

Science made incredible breakthroughs in the last century. Now we can transplant a human heart and grow a human ear on a mouse. Yet we die in vast numbers from awful diseases such as cancer, AIDS, and Alzheimer's.

Our blind faith in modern medicine is reminiscent of Lennie in John Steinbeck's classic novel **Of Mice and Men**, *who was so grateful to his companion George for saving him from drowning that he forgot it was George who had pushed him into the water in the first place!*

Nature has provided us with the most effective protection from disease on Earth: our immune system. Taking drugs destroys it. By allowing our intelligence to act against Nature, we have put evolution into reverse.

Wild animals don't suffer from the huge variety of diseases that we do because they follow Nature's Guide.

THE FLAW IN THE MACHINE

The human being is an incredible machine, infinitely more complex than the car. And yet there is a flaw that has caused us untold misery.

The essential difference between us and wild animals is that they lead their lives instinctively.

We have instincts too, but our intelligence gets in the way. This facility to learn, develop ideas, and communicate has set us apart from the rest of the animal kingdom. It has also given us the impression that we are in control of our own destiny. In fact, our instinct and our intellect are often at odds. This is the flaw in the human machine.

As instinct is an uncalculated response, we don't really understand or trust it. When our instinct and intellect are in conflict, we find it easier to make a decision based on reasoned argument.

Because we don't understand our instincts, we think it's guesswork. But instinct is not hit and miss, it's the result of three billion years of trial and error.

It's what enables wild animals to distinguish between food and poison. Wild animals don't need doctors or hospitals to give birth. Nature is their guide.

I explained that, since humans designed the car, they are the experts on how to maintain it in the best possible condition. It's clear that Nature, not humans, is the leading authority on our bodies. So if your body develops a fault, the logical source to turn to for the solution is Nature's Guide—instinct. You're now ready for the fourth instruction:

IF SOMEONE GIVES YOU ADVICE THAT CONTRADICTS THE ADVICE OF NATURE, REGARDLESS OF HOW EMINENT OR QUALIFIED THAT PERSON MAY BE, IGNORE IT!

FOOD OR POISON?

Wild animals are much more selective than we are about the food they eat and they don't suffer from constipation, diarrhoea, heartburn, indigestion, stomach ulcers, irritable bowel syndrome, high blood pressure, high cholesterol, nor diseases of the stomach, bowel, kidneys, or liver, nor from any of the other degenerative diseases common to humans.

The obvious conclusion is that these conditions are the direct result of our eating habits. Just as a car manufacturer knows best about the fuel and maintenance that a particular car requires, so Nature knows better than we do about the best way to eat.

We will concentrate on understanding Nature's Guide and learning to enjoy following it so that, like wild animals, you will be your ideal weight naturally and effortlessly.

SUMMARY

- **Your body is infinitely more complex than any machine.**
- **Humans designed the car; they didn't design themselves.**
- **The real expert on how your body works is Nature.**
- **Trusting intelligence over instinct has brought us misery.**
- **Ignore any advice that goes against Nature.**

Top Tip No.4

Nature's Guide

Humans ate well and stayed healthy for millions of years without the help of nutritionists or dieticians. So-called experts in the modern world have produced countless guidelines and rules designed to counteract the effects of junk. If they contradict the real expert, Nature, ignore them. Learn to follow the instincts of your mind and body, and live as Nature intended.

CHAPTER 5

YOUR IDEAL WEIGHT

IN THIS CHAPTER
• *A PRECONCEIVED TARGET WEIGHT* • *SEEING IS BELIEVING*
• *YOUR PROBLEM IS SOLVED THE MOMENT YOU UNDERSTAND
THE METHOD* • *THE FIFTH AND SIXTH INSTRUCTIONS*

HOW DO YOU KNOW WHAT YOUR IDEAL WEIGHT IS?

You may well have a specific weight in mind. There's no shortage of weight charts that will tell you. All you need is your height and sex. If you've decided on a target weight this way, please forget it. You have mistakenly put your faith in a guesstimate made by humans. Instead refer to Nature's Guide

ALLEN CARR'S EASYWAY CLINICS

At our weight clinics, it's always interesting when we ask the group to guess the weight of the fastest man on Earth—currently Usain Bolt, the phenomenal Jamaican sprinter. The guesses vary by as much as 50 pounds. If you're expecting me to tell you the actual weight of Usain Bolt, I'm sorry to disappoint you. I have no idea how much he weighs. I have no need to know. It's glaringly obvious that he's in superb physical condition. If you were in a similar physical condition, do you think you'd care how much you weighed?

The fact that these guesses vary by 50 pounds indicates how random setting yourself a target weight is. It shows that we actually have no idea about the correlation between what the scales tell us and what we see when we look in the mirror.

Look at your friends. Do you need a set of scales to decide which of them are overweight and which are not? Of course you don't. Did you come to the conclusion that you're overweight by jumping on the scales? Or was it the sight of your reflection in the mirror; or the fact that your clothes started to feel too tight; or that you felt short of energy and the slightest exertion left you out of breath?

Uncharted territory

The simple equation used by weight charts can only give a ball park figure for your ideal weight. Although there is clearly a relationship between height and weight, it's far from exact.

With my method, you're not going to starve yourself to reach a figure thrown out by a calculator. You're going to achieve your ideal weight by eating your way to health.

Your scales won't tell you when you're the exact weight you want to be, your eyes and your lungs will. If you start out with a preconceived target weight, you're letting the tail wag the dog and creating unnecessary difficulties for yourself. I accept that any weight loss method would be frustrating if you never knew when you had succeeded. I expect you want me to tell you for certain the exact weight you should be. I'm delighted to tell you I can.

Your ideal weight is the weight you happen to be when you can look at yourself naked in a full-length mirror and be happy with your shape. It's the weight you are when you wake up bursting with energy and looking forward to each new day with confidence and joy. It's not a weight decided by trendy magazines and it has nothing to do with equations or guesswork. Allen Carr's Easyway works according to the simple principles of Nature. Your fifth instruction is also very simple:

DON'T START OFF WITH A PRECONCEIVED TARGET WEIGHT

Ponder that last paragraph again: admiring your reflection in the mirror; waking up full of energy; feeling confident and excited about the new day. Anyone of any age can enjoy feeling that way about themselves.

There may be things about your looks you wish were different: a different nose, perhaps, or bigger eyes. I can't do anything about those, but I can promise that you'll radiate health, confidence, and happiness, and those are the most attractive features in any person.

You do not need weighing scales to tell you when you've reached your ideal weight. However, please don't assume from this that you should throw your scales away. They will prove useful.

When I found, after following my method, that I could enjoy a five-mile run at the end of a long day at work and feel really great afterwards, I could hardly believe that previously I couldn't climb a flight of stairs without getting out of breath. When I looked back and realized how much weight I'd lost, it was easy to believe. Keeping a regular record of your weight is not the same as setting yourself a target weight. Don't be a slave to the scales, but use them, say, once a week, to monitor your weight and celebrate as the pounds fall off.

The changes that occur in our appearance are usually gradual. If you look at a photograph of yourself ten years ago, you might be surprised at how different you looked.

The same is true of weight gain. The change in shape is imperceptible from one day to the next, so we hardly notice our slide into obesity. We become conditioned to accept it and don't see it as the disease it is. If the extra bulk appeared overnight, we would be shocked.

My method will enable you to achieve dramatic improvements in appearance, fitness, and health, but it's not one of those diets that claims to work overnight. Anything that puts your body through such a rapid transformation is extremely unpleasant, unhealthy, and unsustainable. Allen Carr's Easyway is enjoyable right from the start. The sixth instruction is:

DO NOT DIET

There's another great advantage to not setting yourself a target weight. If you do, you won't feel you've solved your problem until you've hit your target. In the meantime you'll be waiting for the moment of fulfillment.

The belt test

It's great when you find that your clothes no longer fit, not because they're too tight but because they're too loose! A belt becomes a marvelous accessory in these circumstances. Whoever designed the belt couldn't have foreseen how their invention would become my best friend. When I first started losing weight, I had to use the second hole from the end. The belt had nine holes. As I lost weight I found I had to make new holes to keep my pants from falling down! Each hole I made gave me a tremendous high.

As you follow my method, these encouragements are a constant source of joy.

After a farmer sows his seeds, he goes home at the end of the day content that he's done what he needs to insure a healthy crop. He doesn't have to wait until harvest time to feel satisfied.

With my method, you don't have to wait either. You can start enjoying life immediately, content in the knowledge that, simply by following my method, you've already solved your weight problem. The wheels are already in motion. You're not going on a diet, you're simply changing your way of eating because you want to, and that change starts from day one.

SUMMARY

- Do not begin with a preconceived target weight.
- You'll know when you're the weight you want to be.
- The process is easy, painless, and actually enjoyable.
- The sense of achievement starts from day one.

Top Tip No.5

Your Ideal Weight

Think in terms of your shape, not your weight. Your shape—and whether you are happy with it—is the most reliable indicator of your progress and condition.

CHAPTER 6

FUELING UP AND BURNING OFF

THE BALANCING ACT

When it comes to refueling, why do we treat our bodies so differently from our cars?

By realizing that it's counterproductive to set yourself a target weight, you have already made huge progress. All we have to look at now is intake and disposal, and fortunately these are also easy to deal with. Intake is the quantity and type of food you consume. Disposal is the process of burning energy and disposing of waste matter.

Whenever I mention food, please assume I mean food and drink, and whenever I mention eating, assume I mean eating and drinking, unless I make a clear distinction.

Let's begin by asking why we put on weight. I have no doubt you've asked yourself this many times. The answer is simple: The body will gain weight when our intake exceeds our disposal.

Perhaps you've convinced yourself that there are other reasons why you weigh more than you want. I've heard them all: glandular problems, a slow metabolism, a lack of exercise, age. If you focus on these, you will be led astray. I remind you of the importance of having an open mind.

Nothing grows without being fed. Even if, for any reason, you don't need to eat as much as the next person, that doesn't mean you have to deprive yourself of the food you want and they don't. Is it a problem if your neighbor's car consumes more fuel per mile than yours? Of course not. You don't need to worry about the rate at which your body burns energy.

If you follow Nature's Guide and ignore any conflicting advice, you will be able to eat as much as you want and still be your correct weight, regardless of your glands, metabolic rate, how much you exercise, or your age.

Athletes, dancers, and others who make a career out of vigorous exercise certainly look as if weight is not a problem for them, but just because they seem to control their weight, that doesn't mean they don't have weight problems.

The boxer Ricky Hatton is renowned for his overeating. His job demands that he reaches a target weight, but between fights, he hits the junk food, piles on the pounds, and then embarks on a strict regime to get him back to his target weight in time for the next fight. Hatton is very open about this and there are plenty of others in his profession who have exactly the same problem.

Special exercise is not essential to weight loss. When you exercise, you burn off more fuel, which increases your disposal rate. But exercise also makes you hungrier, so you increase your intake.

> **Running man**
>
> *I knew a man who decided to run the London Marathon. He felt the exercise would help him to shed some weight, as well as giving him a sense of achievement. When he began training a year before the run, he weighed 200 pounds.*
>
> *He got up at six every morning so he could run for an hour before work. Twelve months later he ran the London Marathon and completed the course in just over four hours.*
>
> *He was thrilled with his achievement but weighed exactly the same as he had a year ago. For every calorie he had burned off pounding the roads, he had eaten and drunk more than ever before to satisfy his increased hunger. Furthermore, muscle weighs more than fat, so although he was fitter, trimmer, stronger, and healthier, he did not lose weight. As I will explain later, physical exercise plays an important part in the attainment of overall wellbeing but in itself it does not necessarily help you lose weight.*

If a slim figure were dependent on vigorous exercise, wouldn't many wild animals be tremendously fat? Lions spend around 20 hours a day asleep. Wild animals don't have to spend their lives charging about to keep in shape, they simply balance their intake with their disposal.

FILLING UP

Do you know the weight of the average car? I certainly don't. I've never felt the need to find out. All I know is that when I top it up with fuel the weight increases, and as I drive around and burn fuel, the weight drops. I don't pay it any attention.

Would you take your car for a drive to burn off fuel in order to decrease its weight? That would be idiotic, and it's the same as putting ourselves through special exercise in order to burn calories to lose weight.

You might see a flaw in this comparison. When your car runs out of fuel, it stops running. When your body runs out of fuel, it starts to draw on fat reserves and isn't that exactly what we want?

The trouble with this theory is that after exercise you'll be hungry and thirsty and the natural tendency is to eat to replace the energy you've expended. If you try to resist that urge, it will take willpower and you'll feel deprived and miserable. All you're doing is dieting. And diets don't work!

I may have given the impression that I'm not in favor of exercise. This couldn't be further from the truth. Humans were designed to be active. We were originally obliged to go in search of food and escape predators. Our bodies were not supposed to be slouched in front of a screen all day and they function best when we're physically active. Getting our circulation and breathing going not only makes us feel good, it also makes every function in our body operate more efficiently, including digestion. I love exercise because it helps to keep me fit, toned, healthy, and happy.

Unlike the car, humans did not design the human body and in our efforts to master our understanding of how it works, we've created a fog of confusing misinformation. It's time to simplify and clarify the situation by going back to Nature's Guide.

> ••• **FACT BOX** •••
>
> Today, more people in the world are suffering from obesity than from starvation.

WHY, WHEN, AND WHAT DO WE EAT?

When you sit down to eat, do you think to yourself, "I must eat this food to prevent myself from starving to death?" How many of us actually know what starvation feels like? I was once seriously concerned that I might die through lack of water, but I don't think a day has gone by when I haven't been fortunate enough to have something to eat.

Although avoiding starvation is the ultimate purpose of eating, isn't it true that each meal is prompted by a more immediate reason, such as "I'm in the habit of eating three meals a day," "I enjoy eating," or "Because I got a whiff of something that smelled good," or simply, "The food was there, so I ate it."

Boredom and restlessness are other reasons commonly put forward for eating. They are also common reasons given for smoking. You want some relief, so you reach for the cookies, potato chips, a chocolate bar or a cigarette. But snacking or smoking doesn't relieve boredom or restlessness.

Comfort eating

Boredom and restlessness are usually caused by a problem, be it a piece of work that's proving difficult or a coming event about which we're feeling insecure.

Whatever the problem, it's not hunger. Yet we often reach for a snack in order to comfort ourselves.

How did we come to believe that a problem that has nothing to do with hunger can be solved by eating?

Because that's exactly how snacks have been sold to us by marketing experts.

"Need to make the kids happy? Give them some candy." Does this really make them happy?

"Watching a tense drama, a movie or a football game? Eat some potato chips or popcorn." Does it really improve the experience?

"Want to impress your girlfriends? Give them some fancy chocolate." Does this make them love you more?

If we think we can alleviate boredom and nervousness by eating, why don't we think we could do the same by quenching our thirst?

Most of us eat according to a set routine: three meals a day, morning, noon, and evening. There's nothing wrong with that, in fact it's eminently sensible. But if we eat the same amount regardless of how much energy we've expended, isn't that the same as putting 30 gallons of fuel in your car every week, regardless of how much driving you've done?

If you don't use the car one week, do you still put your usual amount in the tank? There would be fuel spilling out all over the forecourt if you did.

In Nature, hunger is the sign that tells us when we need fuel. This is exactly how wild animals eat. The squirrel knew when to stop eating nuts because it was no longer hungry. We are designed to work in the same way, yet we've become so confused that we let the tail wag the dog. We pump in fuel even when our tank is already full.

> *If we overfill our car, the fuel splashes on to the forecourt. Imagine if it flowed out of the tank and into the engine and trunk. That's effectively what happens with our bodies. For reasons I will explain later, the human body doesn't offload all the excess fuel we pump into it. The junk sloshes into our midriff, buttocks, waist, chest, arms, legs, neck, and face and stays there in unsightly bulges.*

All you have to do is apply the same approach to eating as you do to filling your car. That's what wild animals do. They don't worry about their weight, or how they dispose of the food once they've digested it. All they need to do is supply their bodies with appropriate quantities of their favorite foods. Overeating is caused by eating the wrong foods, i.e. incorrect intake, and this is what lies at the root of your weight problem. It should now be clear that efficiently disposing of what you eat and reaching your ideal weight will happen automatically when you're eating according to Nature's Guide. Most importantly, if you follow my method, you'll find the whole process easy and immensely enjoyable.

SUMMARY

- We gain weight when our intake exceeds our disposal.
- Exercising to burn calories is like driving to burn gasoline.
- Weight and disposal will take care of themselves if intake is correct.

Top Tip No.6

Take a Stroll

Cars are supposed to make life easier, giving us greater freedom and convenience. It's hard to believe when you're sitting waiting outside a supermarket parking lot, or driving around and around the block looking for a parking space. If the supermarket's within walking distance, try leaving your car at home and going on foot, or try shopping little and often at local farmers' markets and grocery stores—it's far more relaxing.

CHAPTER 7

WHAT'S ON THE MENU?

PUTTING DIESEL IN A FERRARI

We need to understand the effects of eating certain types of food

You may be thinking, "All you're saying, Allen, is that I eat too much of the wrong foods. I could have told you that!" That may be the case, but at this stage I'm making no assumptions about the quantity or type of food you eat, I'm simply clarifying that you might well have been confused by having a preconceived idea of what weight you should be aiming for, or by thinking that if you were to exercise more, your problem would be solved. It's important that you erase both these misconceptions from your mind and understand that intake is the critical factor.

It's also important that you're clear about the effect that incorrect intake has on your body. Don't worry, I'm not going to try and frighten you with gory details about the damage that processed foods do to your insides and how eating too much of the wrong foods can cause heart disease, high blood pressure, diabetes, cancer, and obesity, not to mention heartburn, constipation, diarrhoea, stiff joints, tooth decay and bad skin.

Perhaps you fear this is the point where I say you have to give up all your favourite foods. Don't panic. Remember with my method you can:

Eat as much of your favourite foods as you want, whenever you want, as often as you want, and be the exact weight you want to be, without dieting, special exercise, using willpower, or feeling deprived

But you are right about one thing: This is the moment of truth. Now we're dealing with intake, we've reached the point that will determine whether you succeed. If that sounds daunting, remember: Easyway is easy and enjoyable. You have nothing to fear. You're not going to be deprived of anything. On the contrary, you'll soon be feeling the elation of having solved your weight problem.

In the last chapter I talked about adjusting the amount of fuel you put in your car according to the amount the car is used. Now we're going to look at the type of fuel you choose. You obviously know whether your car runs on gasoline or diesel. I certainly hope so; otherwise the consequences would be disastrous!

You don't need to understand anything about the working principles of the internal combustion engine to be aware that you shouldn't put diesel in a gasoline engine or vice versa. As cars have become more sophisticated, they've become more particular about the type of fuel they consume. The manufacturer tells us what to use and we follow the instructions.

The animal kingdom has evolved on similarly sophisticated lines. Every creature on the planet has its own specific intake requirements and the physical attributes to thrive on that intake.

Why has Nature made things so complicated by having a specific ideal intake for each species? If every species were designed to eat the same foods, the biggest and strongest among them would thrive and the smallest and weakest would die. That in turn would condemn the biggest and strongest to extinction, since they depend on the smallest and weakest to survive. The largest creature on the planet, the blue whale, feeds on one of the smallest, plankton, and without the birds, bees, and other flying insects which pollinate plants, our entire ecosystem would collapse.

Nature's ingenuity means each species has the physical attributes to obtain and enjoy its favorite food. Think about the legs and neck of the giraffe, the trunk of the elephant, the snout of the anteater, the teeth and claws of the lion. Just as all creatures have the physical tools to obtain their food, they also have the internal organs to digest it. For example, the cow has four stomachs.

These developments have not happened overnight; they've evolved over millions of years. No species can evolve fast enough to cope with the changes made by man—not even man himself. That's not a flaw in Nature's plan, it's the consequence of humans thinking they know better.

Growing old painfully

The Baby-Boom generation was supposed to have been the most blessed in history. As teenagers in the sixties they experienced new freedoms, worldwide travel, major developments in technology and medicine, and a revolution in the supply and preparation of food.

While humans seemed to be making such rapid "progress," the supermarket shelves were taking their intake ever further away from what Nature Intended.

Today we learn that the Baby Boomers are more susceptible than previous generations to health problems such as aching joints, asthma, diabetes, strokes, and obesity.

No matter how the car engine evolves, it will always be necessary to feed it the correct fuel. In fact, the more sophisticated it becomes, the more specific that fuel has to be. The same applies to your digestive system. Though we may be evolving all the time and living longer, we still need to feed our digestive system the fuel intended for it.

It's ironic that most people treat their cars with the utmost respect and yet regularly fill their bodies with rubbish. Put diesel in a gasoline engine and it'll stop working immediately, yet we can eat all sorts of garbage and keep going. Everyone knows of a child who has swallowed a plastic toy or a coin without any apparent damage. Some entertainers eat broken glass. One man even ate an entire airplane!

The human body is a truly incredible machine that can withstand an enormous amount of abuse and continue to function. But don't be misled into thinking this means you can consume anything you like without doing yourself damage. Eating the wrong type of food may not stop us in our tracks, as diesel will stop a gasoline car, but it does have disastrous consequences. If we don't eat the food that Nature has designed for us, we become fat, slow, and lethargic until we finally grind to a halt.

The gasoline engine contaminated with diesel has to be flushed through at great expense to work again. Your body pushes anything it's not designed to digest into out-of-the-way places. These toxins gather as unsightly fat deposits, clogging up your bloodstream and suffocating your entire body.

THE NATURAL CHOICE

Animals don't have these problems because they eat only natural foods. By that I mean food that is eaten in its natural state. Not refined, frozen, pickled, preserved, smoked, sweetened, flavored, fermented, mixed, added to, or cooked.

Maybe alarm bells are ringing. "Are you telling me I'm no longer allowed to cook?" No, I'm saying nothing of the sort.

REMEMBER, WITH MY METHOD THERE ARE NO RESTRICTIONS

Earlier I emphasized the importance of an open mind. So discard your preconceptions and think about the foods that would be available to you if you followed the example of wild animals. I'm talking about foods that require no cooking or processing yet taste wonderful without any need for flavorings, seasoning, or sauces.

Do you agree that it comes down to fruit, vegetables, nuts, and seeds? Apart from these, even the most basic of everyday foods has been tampered with. When you come home and you want a quick snack, you might opt for some bread and jam. It seems natural enough, but let's look closely at the manufacturing process and ingredients.

Starting with the bread: a mixture of milled and refined flour, yeast, salt, and numerous additives, baked at high temperature. Now the butter: cow's milk pasteurized, homogenized, churned, and refrigerated to prevent it from decomposing. The jam is made by boiling the life out of fruit and adding refined sugar and preservatives.

You might argue that all this tampering is for the better, improving the foods in question. But does it really improve them? Or does it simply kill any natural goodness or nutritional value the ingredients had to begin with?

Cooking food destroys vital vitamins, antioxidants, and essential fatty acids. However, you can carry on cooking delicious meals, and you don't have to restrict yourself to fresh fruit, vegetables, nuts, and seeds. My method restores the joy of eating and makes it easy for you to attain your ideal weight.

If you were happy eating just fresh fruit, vegetables, nuts, and seeds, you would enjoy a very healthy and energetic life, free from weight problems. But Nature's ingenious design has a built-in margin for error, which means we can eat a certain amount of "second-rate" foods without causing problems. I will explain more about this "Junk Margin" later. For now, I want you to be reassured that my method is not about forbidding certain foods.

This margin for error is different for all species. The koala bear is limited exclusively to eucalyptus leaves, whereas the goat can survive on almost anything. However, no other species on the planet can match the variety of food eaten by humans. Because of our intellect, we've ended up eating a uniquely varied and processed selection of foods.

Not only are we able to eat meat, vegetables, fruit, and fish, we even tend to combine this variety of foods within the same meal, even in the same mouthful. Indeed many people feel that unless they have their "meat and two vegetables" at each meal, they've been shortchanged. Our stomachs try to cope with this wide range of foods, but the very fact that you're reading this book tells us that it's not a recipe for slimness, health, or happiness.

You can't just put any old food in your mouth and expect your digestive system to get on with it. What if your car ran out of gas miles from the nearest garage and I told you, "Don't worry, your car runs on gasoline, which is made from crude oil. There's a plastic bag in your boot. Plastic also happens to be made from crude oil. We can stuff it into the gas tank. That should do the trick."

It's clearly a ridiculous suggestion and you'd probably wonder if I'd gone crazy, but we, and so-called expert nutritionists, apply the same illogical principle to our bodies. I call it "the Plastic Bag Syndrome," and we're going to explore it in the next chapter.

SUMMARY

- Understand the effects of eating the wrong foods.
- All animals are designed to eat foods specific to them.
- I'm not imposing restrictions. There's also a Junk Margin.

Top Tip No. 7

Start with a Salad

Natural foods make you feel best. Make sure you have some raw, natural, unprocessed food at every meal. Start lunch and dinner with a salad. Mix as many raw vegetables as you want. Cover your plate in color: red tomatoes, green lettuce, and yellow peppers. Grate raw carrot and beets. Good-quality extra virgin olive oil and lemon juice will dress your food perfectly.

CHAPTER 8

THE PLASTIC BAG
SYNDROME

IN THIS CHAPTER
- *WHERE DO WE GET OUR NUTRIENTS?*
- *THE CONSEQUENCES OF EATING JUNK*
- *THE DIGESTIVE PROCESS*

THERE'S NO SUBSTITUTE FOR QUALITY

If we eat meat for protein, why not eat teeth for calcium? The fact that something contains nutrients we need doesn't necessarily make that food suitable for us to eat

Put something other than the recommended fuel in your car's tank and you could cause serious damage to the engine. But you can always replace your car. You only get one body.

You would think that would make us look after our bodies infinitely more carefully than we look after our cars. Yet the reality is that we treat them more like a waste disposal unit.

Perhaps you believe this is one of the many advantages of being a human being. After all, the giant panda and the koala bear are under threat because they eat only one plant. I have news for you. Humans as a whole may not be under immediate threat of extinction, but each individual consuming this incredible variety of food invites obesity, disease, and premature death.

We're not very discriminating about food. So long as something is edible and not classed as a poison we regard it as food. We eat it without a second thought as to how our digestive system is going to cope.

Would you eat a piece of chalk or an iron nail? Unless you're a circus act like Monsieur Mangetout, aka Michel Lotto—the Frenchman who once ate an entire airplane—I think I'm safe in assuming you would not. But why not? After all, we've been told by so-called experts that we need calcium and iron for healthy bones and blood. We also need protein, and meat is high in protein, so they tell us to eat the flesh of animals and convince us that if we don't, we risk suffering a protein deficiency.

Have you ever stopped to wonder where those animals get their protein from? Have you ever seen a cow feeding on the flesh of another animal? Cows are considerably bigger and stronger than us. They eat no meat at all. Neither, for that matter, do elephants, rhinoceroses, giraffes, hippopotamuses, horses, buffalo, gorillas… the list is virtually endless. The largest and strongest animals on land are all herbivores.

We need protein to build muscle, so we're told to eat meat. This is the Plastic Bag Syndrome. If we follow that logic, shouldn't we eat teeth and bones too, in order to get calcium? Or simpler still, a piece of chalk? Instead, we're advised to eat cheese and drink milk to obtain calcium.

How much cheese does an elephant eat? How much milk does it drink? I've never seen any teeth larger than the tusks of an elephant—and all that without a single morsel of cheese. The fact is, an elephant gets all the protein and calcium it needs by eating only vegetation.

I can sense the meat eaters among you feeling uneasy at this point. "Allen's going to try and turn me into a vegetarian." Remember with my method you can:

Eat as much of your favorite foods as you want, whenever you want, as often as you want, and be the exact weight you want to be without dieting, special exercise, using willpower, or feeling deprived

I'm certainly not about to insist you go on a diet of any kind, vegetarian or otherwise. I'm simply explaining the false logic in the advice we're given by so-called experts such as doctors and nutritionists.

The food we eat passes through a highly sophisticated process we call digestion. It begins at the chewing stage, where saliva mixes with the food in the mouth and starts to break it down. Once the food reaches the stomach, the digestive juices come into play, breaking it down further. The stomach adjusts its digestive juices according to what we eat. When it's done its best, the food travels into the intestines where the nutrients are extracted and distributed around the body, and the remaining waste matter is then disposed of via the colon.

This last part of the process can only take place effectively if the food has been properly digested. You can insure this happens by eating in its natural state the food that Nature has provided,

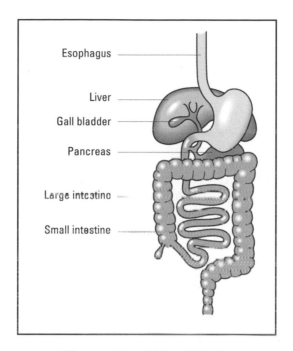

Esophagus

Liver

Gall bladder

Pancreas

Large intestine

Small intestine

Like an engine, with the right fuel our
digestive system operates efficiently

and by being active enough to insure that your metabolism is
ticking over efficiently. If you don't, your body will not function
properly and this will lead to weight problems.

Until now you may have tried focusing on counting calories,
taking supplements, avoiding carbohydrates, etc. That takes the
joy out of eating. Now you can stop worrying about such details.
Nature's Guide automatically insures you get everything you
need in exactly the right balance.

The wrong advice is part of the brainwashing. I will help you
to unravel the brainwashing and follow your instincts.

There's a close relationship between you and your body. Your body will look after you IF you look after your body. It's a partnership. Fail to fulfill your end of the deal and you can hardly complain if your body gives up on you.

Understanding the consequences

It's not necessary to know how your car works in order to keep it running properly. Nor is it necessary to know how your digestive system works in order to keep your body running properly, provided you follow Nature's Guide. However, I want you to understand the basics of digestion so that you can see clearly what happens if you don't follow the Guide.

I used to be a chain smoker and was well aware of the risk of lung cancer, but it didn't make me quit. I hoped that I would be one of the lucky ones who escaped the disease and thought that if I did, I would get away scot-free. It was like Russian roulette. You either got lung cancer or you didn't. I ignored the huge damage that smoking was doing to my insides, the coagulation of my blood, the blocking of my veins and arteries, and the terrible strain put on my heart as it tried to keep the thickening gunge circulating through my system.

For the first 50 years of my life I took the same attitude to eating as I did to smoking. I buried my head in the sand and told myself that I was just one of those people who preferred to live life to the full and die young, rather than live like a monk to a grand old age. Live life to the full? How could I be so blind? I was overweight, lethargic, and short of breath. I suffered from regular bouts of indigestion and constipation. When I gave in to temptation, I felt guilty. When I resisted, I felt deprived.

Once I had learned a bit about how digestion works, I was amazed that indigestion, heartburn, and constipation were all I had suffered. It made me aware of the incredible job that our bodies do in withstanding the abuse that we subject them to every day, year after year.

We know our body is irreplaceable. So why do we destroy it? We're not stupid; our intelligence is what sets us above every other animal on the planet. The only explanation has to be that we don't realize what we're doing because we're shrouded in ignorance and confusion.

The car manufacturer's guide makes caring for your car very simple. But when it comes to eating, we're expected to find the instructions in a whole library of guides, all offering conflicting messages based on a mishmash of tradition, ignorance, advertising, and convenience. The outcome is confusion. Nature's Guide makes caring for your body very simple.

So how do we learn when and what to eat to attain our ideal weight and be fit and healthy without feeling deprived? It was a marvelous moment when I discovered that it's all in Nature's Guide.

I wish I'd found out sooner, but I now know it's never too late. Fortunately for you, you don't have to work it out for yourself. Once you counter the brainwashing, all will come naturally. My method will show you the way.

-------------------- **SUMMARY** --------------------
- You only get one body. Look after it.
- The strongest animals on earth don't get their protein from meat.
- To get the nutrients we need from food, it must be properly digestible. Don't put plastic bags in your fuel tank!
- Nature's Guide takes care of all your nutritional needs.

Top Tip No.8

The Right Stuff

You won't need extra vitamins or supplements. All your nutritional needs can be taken care of by eating the right foods. They have everything we need to give us the strength and energy to live life to the full. You will no longer be overweight or lethargic as your body will be functioning efficiently.

CHAPTER 9

TRUST YOUR SENSES

IN THIS CHAPTER
• *HOW YOUR SENSOR DECIDES WHAT'S GOOD TO EAT*
• *THE SIXTH SENSE*
• *REMOVING THE MENTAL TUG-OF-WAR*

LOSING OUR WAY

Nature's Guide insures that all wild animals love to eat the foods that keep them fit, healthy, and the ideal weight. Why do humans stray?

How do we distinguish between food and poison and how do we know which are the best foods for us? Parents go out of their way to make sure that poisons are kept away from their children. We print labels on poisons: "toxic," "keep out of the reach of children," "not to be taken internally," etc.

We don't have to use our own judgment, we're taught not to consume poisons. How do wild animals know? They can't put labels on things or tell each other what to avoid. And how have they learned what are the best foods for them?

All creatures have a Sensor designed to tell them what to eat and what not to eat. Using sight, smell, hearing, touch, and taste, they can establish whether something is edible and whether it's the type of food for them. Watch an animal when it approaches unfamiliar food. It won't dive in like we do and start munching away. First it will scrutinize the food, perhaps circling it once or twice. Then it will sniff it. If the food passes these tests, the animal will touch it suspiciously, always ready to walk away. And finally it will taste it, taking a small morsel to test before tucking into the rest.

This is how Nature enables all animals to detect the best food for them. These senses are all any animal needs. It's an ingenious system and it works like a dream. So why doesn't it work for us? Why do so many things that are bad for us, like cakes, chocolate, ice cream, candy, and alcohol, seem so appealing to our senses? Why didn't she apply the same logic to human beings and make the things that are bad for us taste foul and the things that are good for us taste fantastic? I'm delighted to tell you that's exactly what she did.

We are designed to know our favorite foods through our Sensor. It's the practical instrument that interprets and puts to use Nature's Guide to insure that we are at our optimum in body and mind: fit, healthy, and the ideal weight.

In the modern age the speed with which we spread information is matched by the speed with which we spread misinformation. Humans believe that poisons give them pleasure because they've been brainwashed. Their Sensor has been overridden. We're led to believe that things like oysters, which look, feel, smell, and taste awful, are a delicacy. Once we remove the brainwashing, our Sensor takes charge again and the truth stands out bright and clear:

THE FOODS THAT TASTE BEST ARE THE BEST FOR YOU

The cat's whiskers

Even though she's grown up being fed by humans, my cat still trusts her own senses when it comes to food. I've often watched her go through her rigmarole: first eyeing up the food; then sniffing it, touching it, and finally tasting a morsel. She then either tucks in or walks haughtily away with her tail in the air, as if the new gourmet cat food I've bought for her were poison. Cats can be very full of airs and graces at times.

She should be grateful. I didn't choose her, she chose me. She just strayed into our house one day and decided to stay. I've been feeding her ever since. Of course it was silly to get infuriated by a cat's ingratitude. How was she to know that the cat food company and I were only doing what was best for her?

Yes, I actually believed that a cat food manufacturer knew better than my cat what her favorite food was. How stupid! How arrogant! I'm grateful to my cat for drawing my attention to the mistake.

These days we put "sell by," "use by," and "best before" dates on food. Wild animals don't need these because their Sensor does it for them. As a natural food goes off, it changes in look, smell, and feel, repulsing the senses that were previously attracted to it.

Let's take an apple: That shiny, taut skin turns brown and speckled with mold; the sweet, delicate smell turns acrid and strong; the crisp flesh becomes soft and mushy. It will taste foul too, but you don't need to go that far. Your other senses will have already warned you off. On the rare occasions that your Sensor overlooks something poisonous, your digestive system will do everything it can to eject the poison by vomiting or diarrhoea.

It's hard to comprehend how Nature devised such a sophisticated system and until I became intrigued by a squirrel one day, I didn't even realize it had. Thanks to that squirrel, I realized that I had spent the first 50 years of my life overriding my Sensor. The beautiful truth is:

THE FOODS THAT ARE BEST FOR YOU TASTE AND SMELL GOOD. POISONS TASTE AND SMELL AWFUL

Sense and sensibility

Taste is the strongest indication we have that something is not good for us to eat, and the other senses play a part too. Smell is very closely linked to taste. You may have noticed how all food becomes tasteless when your nose is blocked. Appearance and texture are strong indicators too. Ask any chef about the importance of presentation. It doesn't just apply to prepared food: Natural foods also attract or repel us according to their look and feel. A good chef looks at, feels, and smells the food he's buying to make sure he selects the best ingredients. If any of our senses rejects a food, we should take heed. Think about the suspicion with which an animal approaches food. I'm not saying you have to approach every meal with suspicion, but you do need to learn to trust your senses and unlock the knowledge you have inside your body.

We sometimes talk about a sixth sense. You look up and down the road and see no traffic, but as you go to step off the curb, something holds you back. At that moment a car goes by, a car you were sure wasn't there. Your sixth sense has saved you. Sometimes we look but don't see, listen but don't hear, touch but don't feel. If one sense fails, the others step in. You didn't see the car, but perhaps you heard it, though you failed to register the fact consciously. Your intellect told you it was safe to cross the road, but your instinct knew it wasn't. Instinct is the result of three billion years of natural logic, it's the greatest knowledge there is. Without instinct, no creatures would survive.

Once we've gotten rid of the brainwashing with my method, you will be able to solve your weight problem without experiencing any conflict between your mind and your senses and you won't need to use willpower. With the help of natural logic, instinct, and Nature's Guide, the uncertainty and confusion disappear because you know that the foods that keep you slim, fit, and healthy are also the foods that taste the best: your favorite foods.

One of the worst things about having a weight problem is the schizophrenia, the tug-of-war in our mind between two conflicting voices. On one hand, "I would love to be slim, fit, and healthy." On the other, "Boy, would I love that cream cake." We're going to remove one side of this tug-of-war, leaving you free to be your ideal weight without a struggle.

You're probably itching to find out exactly which foods are recommended in the Guide. Please be patient, we will come to that very soon. First there are other aspects to the Guide that you need to understand. Remember how the squirrel knew when to stop eating the nuts. Nature's Guide doesn't just tell us what to eat, it also tells us when to eat and how much. Remember, you will be able to eat as much of your favorite foods as you want, whenever you want, as often as you want. Let's see how.

------------------------ **SUMMARY** ------------------------
- **Our Sensor tells us which foods to eat.**
- **Foods that taste the best are the best for you.**
- **The belief that junk tastes good is an illusion, the result of brainwashing.**
- **If one of your senses rejects a food, take heed!**
- **The sixth sense is the result of three billion years of logic.**

Top Tip No.9

Your Sensor

Once you've got rid of the brainwashing, you'll be able to use your Sensor to distinguish between right and wrong foods. It's a natural process. Your taste buds will be attracted to the foods that are best for you: your favorite foods. There's nobody who can guide you better than your own body. It knows what it needs. When it's happy, it can help you to enjoy life. When it's overworked by eating junk, you suffer from indigestion, heartburn, constipation, and obesity.

CHAPTER 10

WHEN TO EAT

IN THIS CHAPTER
• WHY HUNGER IS GOOD • HUNGER AND YOUR SENSOR
• SATISFYING YOUR HUNGER • READING NATURE'S GAUGE
• THE SEVENTH INSTRUCTION

ENJOYING EATING

We need to eat. This is why Nature designed eating to be such a pleasurable experience

At Allen Carr's Easyway clinics we ask clients why they eat. Their replies include: "to beat boredom," "to relieve stress," "to comfort myself," "to give myself a reward," or "just following routine." Remarkably, it always takes a while before anybody mentions the one true reason for eating.

You refuel your car when the fuel gauge tells you you're running low. You would think Nature would have come up with something that did the same job for us. The beautiful truth is, it did: hunger. The problem is we don't use it. As babies we know when to stop feeding. Our Gauge tells us when we're no longer hungry. As we grow up, we're brainwashed by society to lose touch with our hunger.

Imagine if you had created something as amazing as the

animal kingdom. You've given them all these ingenious senses that enable them to determine which foods they should eat. How do you make sure they eat them in the right quantity and at the right times? Hunger is what tells wild animals when they need to refuel and hunger is our true reason for eating.

The word "hunger" has strong connotations. We associate it with famine and disturbing pictures of starving children in poor countries. In fact, hunger is not a problem; it's the inability to satisfy hunger that's the problem. Hunger is essential to the enjoyment of eating.

We have a tendency to exaggerate. "I'm starving" is a common way of saying we feel hungry. If you had ever experienced real starvation, I doubt you would use the word so lightly.

Feeling hungry?

Most people eat three meals a day, one in the morning, one around the middle of the day, and one in the evening. People use different terms to describe these meals. I will call them breakfast, lunch, and dinner.

If we miss lunch, we may say we're "starving" by the time it comes to dinner, but in reality we're in no pain. In fact if we forget to have lunch, we may not even notice until later in the day. Hunger signals will start to flow to our brains during the day as the fuel we've consumed at breakfast is gradually burned off, yet we needn't suffer any discomfort.

There were several pieces of evidence that led me to discover the secret of being the right weight. The first was seeing the squirrel stop eating the nuts and start storing them. The second was the realization that hunger is not a pain to be feared but an ingenious device which insures our survival by telling us when and how much to eat, thereby giving us pleasure at every meal.

It's important to understand that hunger is not to be feared. Satisfying our hunger is one of the greatest pleasures in life and, provided you follow Nature's Guide and all of my instructions, it's one you can enjoy every day for the rest of your life.

HUNGER AND THE SENSOR

Perhaps you're familiar with the French expression "bon appetit." The reason the French wish you a "good appetite" is because they know that the greater your hunger, the more you'll enjoy the meal. They recognize that there's a direct connection between hunger and taste.

In Chapter 9 we learned that we have a Sensor—a combination of our five senses—that tells us what is the best food for us. This Sensor also plays a major role in telling us when we're hungry and when and how much to eat.

You will have experienced this for yourself. I once ordered some Chinese food from room service in a hotel. It looked, smelled, and tasted delicious but was too much to finish. When I returned from a walk later, the food was still there, but now the look and smell had lost their charm and I had no desire to taste it.

In fact, I didn't have another Chinese meal for months.

Food only tastes good if you're hungry. Indeed, the hungrier you get, the readier your tastebuds are to enjoy a range of foods. In James Clavell's novel *King Rat*, about American and English POWs in Singapore during World War II, the prisoners developed a taste for rats, breeding them for meat. This illustrates how extreme hunger will give us a taste for foods we would otherwise find disgusting.

The real pleasure in eating is the satisfaction of your hunger. You may dispute this. After all, do we not take great pleasure in the ritual that surrounds eating? Whether it's a meal out in a restaurant with friends, or a dinner party at home that gives us an excuse to lay the table with our best china, some of the best social occasions are centered on eating. Yes, but if there were no food, do you think you would still enjoy the ritual? Of course we can enjoy social occasions without eating, but not if we're hungry. It's also true that we will only enjoy eating when we're hungry. Of course we prefer to end our hunger with our favorite foods, but if you carry on eating them after you're full, they will no longer taste good, you will cease to enjoy them and feel sick. Furthermore, as we've seen from *King Rat*, if you're hungry enough, even a rat will become a delicacy.

Sex was designed to give us pleasure so that we reproduce and insure the survival of the species. Eating was designed to give us pleasure so we survive as individuals. We've been brainwashed into believing there's pleasure in eating purely for eating's sake. But you will only enjoy eating if you're hungry, so the real pleasure lies in satisfying your hunger. The senses, or our Sensor, identify our favorite foods. Our nostrils are filled with lovely aromas; our eyes feast on the colors and textures on our plate; and our taste buds are aroused as the food touches our tongue. All this adds to the pleasure of ending our hunger. If you follow Nature's Guide and consume the right foods at the right time in the right quantity, eating will become the great pleasure it's designed to be and you will find it easy and enjoyable to be your ideal weight.

READING NATURE'S GAUGE

Hunger is the gauge Nature has given us to measure our need for food. So when exactly should we eat?

It's important to avoid mistaking other feelings for hunger. This will become easier as you follow my method and get back in touch with your body. I mentioned that clients at our clinics say they eat for all sorts of reasons including comfort and stress relief. The empty, insecure feeling of hunger feels the same as normal stress. You know that feeling you get in the pit of your stomach when you get worrying news, or you're late for an important appointment, or you nearly drive into the car in front. Stress may feel the same as hunger, but food does not relieve it.

IF YOU'RE BORED OR NEED TO BE COMFORTED, DON'T RUSH TO THE FRIDGE. REMEMBER, IF YOU'RE NOT HUNGRY, EATING WON'T HELP.

Beware of foods advertised on television. They're encouraging you to eat when you're not hungry and the food is almost certainly not in Nature's Guide. Learn to recognize when you're hungry. Realize that hunger pangs are very slight and pass very quickly even if you don't eat. So if you feel a little hunger pang, don't panic if it's not convenient to eat at that moment. On the contrary, look forward to satisfying that hunger at your next meal. Remember, hunger is your friend, not your enemy. It enables you to enjoy the marvelous pleasure of eating. If you find yourself feeling hungry at unexpected times, ask yourself whether it's actually hunger or something else. Ask yourself the following questions: When did I last eat? Has something just happened which could be causing me stress? Is it just boredom? Trying to satisfy any feeling other than hunger by eating will make you bloated, fat, more stressed, and miserable.

My seventh instruction is:

ONLY EAT WHEN YOU'RE HUNGRY

SUMMARY

- Hunger is the one true reason for eating.
- See hunger as a source of pleasure.
- The hungrier you are, the better food will taste.
- Hunger involves no physical pain.
- The true pleasure to be derived from eating is the satisfying of hunger.
- Avoid eating unless you're hungry.

Top Tip No.10

Satisfying your Hunger

Eat slowly. As you enjoy each mouthful think about the nutritional value and the taste of the food. Value the goodness you're putting into your body and be aware of the feeling of satisfaction. There's no reason to overeat. You will be receiving immense pleasure from your food several times a day. There's no reason to continue once your hunger's satisfied. There's no pleasure in overeating. Listen to Nature's Gauge.

CHAPTER 11

WHEN TO STOP EATING

IN THIS CHAPTER
• RECOGNIZING WHEN YOU'RE SATISFIED
• THE IMPORTANCE OF EATING THE RIGHT FOODS • HOW WE'VE BEEN
BRAINWASHED TO OVEREAT • VARIETY • THE JUNK MARGIN

GET BACK IN TOUCH WITH YOUR BODY

The same Gauge that tells you when to eat also tells you when to stop

The problem is that we've been brainwashed to disregard our Gauge. We're constantly bombarded by mixed messages from a variety of sources about when and what we should be eating, and we've lost touch with how to recognize the messages from our own body. Hunger is our friend, not just because it tells us when to eat and enables us to enjoy the process but also because, as soon as it's satisfied, it sends a signal to stop eating, and so stops us overeating.

Overeating makes us bloated and uncomfortable. If our Gauge works, why do we ever feel the desire to overeat? Surely it should send a signal to stop before we go too far.

The greater the proportion of high-water-content foods we eat, the less bloated we feel. High-water-content foods such as fresh fruit and vegetables cleanse the intestines and help us to absorb the essential nutrients. Hunger ends when we've absorbed sufficient nourishment from the right foods, not when we've stuffed ourselves with junk which provides few nutrients and can never truly satisfy the requirements of our bodies. This is why eating the right foods removes the compulsion to overeat.

I may be giving you the impression that you need to go through some sort of meditative ritual in order to reestablish contact with your inner self. I assure you it's far simpler than that. Luckily, Nature's Gauge does the work for you. Once you've consumed sufficient nutrients, it registers "satisfied" and your desire to keep eating ends.

When you drink a glass of water, you stop drinking when your thirst is quenched, not when your belly is full. The same applies to eating—provided you eat the right foods.

When you regularly eat foods that do not contain the required nutrients, overeating becomes the norm. You've overridden the tools supplied by Nature and no longer know how to listen to what they're telling you. Your Sensor has stopped leading you to the right foods and you no longer use your Gauge correctly. You've lost touch with your body and however much you would like to be your ideal weight, you cannot achieve it.

EATING THE WRONG FOODS LEADS TO OVEREATING

Only by eating the right foods will you achieve satisfaction. And only by achieving satisfaction will you feel that your hunger has ended. All you have to do is reverse the brainwashing that has prevented you from recognizing your favorite foods and realizing when you've satisfied your hunger.

A meal to die for

Steak and french fries is many people's favorite meal. I have to admit I used to be rather partial to it myself, particularly at my local steakhouse restaurant which served up huge portions. By the time I'd polished it off, I would be pushing my chair back from the table and loosening my belt. But was I satisfied? When the dessert menu came round, somehow I'd feel the need for a portion of chocolate fudge cake too.

Though the steak and fries had left me feeling uncomfortably full, it hadn't satisfied my real hunger. My Gauge sensed that I had not received the nutrients I needed, and so it did not register "satisfied." Craving satisfaction, I mistakenly ordered the chocolate fudge cake.

The sugar-filled dessert didn't provide the necessary nutrients either and so I'd come to the end of the meal feeling both full and hungry at the same time. I'd been brainwashed into making two misjudgments: first, that steak and fries and chocolate fudge cake were two of my favorite foods; and, second, that the more I ate, the more satisfied I would feel.

HOW MUCH WOULD YOU LIKE?

From an early age we're told that it's wasteful, not to mention insulting to the cook, to leave anything on our plate and so we feel obliged to polish it all off whether we feel truly hungry or not. But who decides how much food is put on your plate? Can the person serving you gauge your hunger better than you?

From the moment we're weaned off the bottle or our mother's breast, the quantity of food we're given at each meal is determined by someone else. Our parents dish up what they consider to be a healthy portion at meal times; go to a restaurant and it's the chef, not you, who decides how much to put on your plate. Who decides how many potato chips go in each package? Who decides how big that chocolate bar should be? No wonder you feel that your eating is out of your control.

Providing you eat the foods Nature intended, knowing when to eat and when to stop is simple: Eat when you're hungry and stop when you're not. Stick to this principle and you'll find that every meal becomes enjoyable and you'll have no weight problems.

Eat slowly and give your body time to register that it's received the nutrients it requires, and you'll find it much easier to sense when to stop. This also allows you time to savor the food and increases the pleasure of eating.

Does the thought of stopping eating before you feel completely stuffed make you feel deprived? Perhaps you think I'm trying to restrict the amount you eat, like a diet. I assure you I'm not. Remember, you can eat as much of your favorite foods as you want. Is it really a restriction to stop eating when you're satisfied? Why would you want to go on eating beyond that point? Do you like being bloated? With my method you'll rediscover the beautiful truth provided by nature:

EATING IS A PLEASURE, OVEREATING IS A PAIN

THE SPICE OF LIFE

You will only be completely satisfied if you eat the right foods. Again I can hear alarm bells ringing. Does this mean you're no longer going to be allowed to enjoy the wide variety of foods that is currently available to you?

In every aspect of our consumer society humans have created a dazzling array of options to tempt us. Take nicotine, for example. You have the choice of how to take it: cigarettes, cigars, pipes, chewing tobacco, snuff, gum, patches, nasal sprays, inhalators, e-cigarettes etc. You can smoke ready-mades or roll ups. You also have countless brands of cigarettes and tobaccos to choose from. This huge variety makes us feel we have a great freedom of choice.

It's the same with alcohol. You can choose beer, wine, or spirits. Perhaps whiskey is your tipple, but which one? There are thousands of brands.

Big Food offers the most choice of all. Isn't it a joy to have so many choices when it comes to mealtimes? Humans appear to have invented an almost infinite number of brands. Take breakfast, for example. There's a huge variety of cereals available to the consumer, marketed in very different ways—though most contain the same ingredients. I wonder how much of this huge variety you incorporate in your regular life.

I have noticed from my work with nicotine addiction that smokers have many quirks, one of the most consistent being their insistence on smoking a particular brand. Despite the thousands of options available to them, they go out of their way to obtain their usual brand. It doesn't bother them that they're not making the most of the variety on offer. In fact, what's more likely to upset them is when they can't get hold of their usual brand, which they've forced their brains and bodies to become accustomed to.

I used to think this was just one of the many idiosyncrasies particular to smokers, but I have since realized that we tend to do the same with food. There are countless different foods to choose from, and yet we stick to the same handful. Next time you shop, count the number of different foods in your basket. Now think how often you vary the items on your shopping list. There may be the odd change from week to week, depending on the weather, your mood, availability, or your budget, but the majority of items will be the same week in, week out.

Nowadays some people do their food shopping online and this highlights how little our purchases vary. The clever computer saves the details of your last shop and all you need to do is press a button to request an identical delivery. Sometimes people remove, add, or change an item, but mostly they stick to the same items and eat the same things week after week.

Your usual, sir?

There may be a great variety of junk available to us, but we certainly don't need it and most of us don't take advantage of it. Two examples from my own experience clearly illustrate this.

Like many people, I used to begin the day with a bowl of cereal. My local supermarket had a whole aisle devoted to the different brands of breakfast cereal, but I still took home the same one every time. Once we've decided on a favorite food, we're happy to eat it time after time.

The second example of this struck me one evening when I was out for a curry. There were a lot of Indian restaurants near my house, and I had my favorite, the Motspur Park Tandoori. As I sat there perusing the menu, the owner, Malik, came over to take my order. The restaurant was unusually busy and he was in a hurry. Before I could say anything, he recited exactly what I had intended to order. How? Because I ordered the same thing every time!

I hadn't even realized it myself. It later struck me that it wasn't just at the Tandoori, it was the same story when I went out for a Chinese or an Italian meal. I would sit poring over the descriptions on the menu, trying to make a decision. And every time I would choose the same dishes that I knew I liked.

We're happy to eat the same foods repeatedly if they're our favorites. Why wouldn't we be? Given a choice between the foods we like most and other options, who in their right mind would choose the alternatives? And there's nothing wrong with that, as long as our favorites provide the energy and nutrients that our body requires and keep us fit and healthy.

Compared to wild animals, we do eat a wide variety of foods. However, we've been brainwashed to eat junk. With my method, you'll still be eating a wide variety, but of your favorite foods.

We've established that only by eating the right foods will you be able to satisfy your hunger completely, and only by doing that will you be able to sense the ideal time to stop. My method will not restrict your choice of foods and you will not be left feeling deprived.

You will eat the foods that you truly enjoy and afterward you will feel fit, healthy, and energetic instead of bloated, sluggish, and guilty.

MARGIN FOR ERROR

Nature has insured that there are ideal foods for each animal and she has also provided second- and third-rate foods in order to insure survival under difficult circumstances. The gorilla, for example, prefers to feed on fruit. But when fruit is not available, it will eat other vegetation to survive. When fruit becomes available the gorilla will revert to it, because fruit is its favorite food—the food that tastes best to the gorilla.

Does the gorilla realize that if it doesn't eat anything it will die and, therefore, make a conscious decision to force down some other vegetation when fruit is unavailable? Or does it move on to other vegetation by instinct? Actually its Sensor is guiding the gorilla to find a way to relieve its hunger. As it grows hungrier and hungrier, its second-rate and third-rate foods taste better and better.

Nature has insured that animals can survive when their favorite foods are unavailable. The gorilla doesn't have to make a conscious decision. Its Sensor and hunger make the decision for it. Since it reverts to its favorite foods as soon as possible, the second- and third-rate foods cause no long-term problems.

This is good news for the gorilla. It's also good news for us. While Nature has provided us with our favorite foods, she has also allowed a liberal margin for error. As long as we consume mainly the foods that were designed for us, we can go on eating junk without causing any serious problems.

This is what I mean by the Junk Margin and it's an essential part of my method. Unlike diets, you never have to think, "I'm not allowed to eat this or that." There are no rigid restrictions and the bulk of what you eat will be the favorite foods Nature intended for you.

At this point I ought to clarify what I mean by junk food. To most people it means fast food, confectionery, cakes, etc.—the sorts of food that nutritionists all tend to agree are bad for us. My definition of junk is anything not in its natural state, anything that has been tampered with.

With the mass production of processed food, eating junk has become the norm for many of us, and our favorite foods have become secondary. With my method we reverse the brainwashing by learning to listen to the natural signals in our body. When you eat your favorite foods, you will sense the good they're doing to your body instead of feeling guilty about the harm caused by junk. Then you can enjoy a feeling of well-being every time you eat.

SUMMARY

- **Your Gauge and your Sensor will tell you when your hunger is satisfied. That's when to stop eating.**
- **A lack of nutrients leads to overeating.**
- **Satisfaction will only be achieved by eating the right foods.**
- **Eat slowly to give the nutrients time to register.**
- **We're brainwashed into overeating.**
- **Understand the Junk Margin.**

Top Tip No. 11

Take your Time

Digestion starts the moment you put food into your mouth. Savor each mouthful and don't rush. Chew slowly and thoroughly, especially when you're eating grains and pulses, and let your saliva start breaking the food down. By eating slowly you will be able to sense your hunger being satisfied, you will enjoy your meals more, and you will know when you've eaten enough.

CHAPTER 12

HOW WE LOST NATURE'S GUIDE

IN THIS CHAPTER

• *ACQUIRED AND UNACQUIRED TASTE* • *THE WARNING LIGHTS*
• *THE PROCESSED FOOD REVOLUTION* • *THE EIGHTH INSTRUCTION*
• *UNDOING THE BRAINWASHING* • *SWEET DECEPTION*

NO SACRIFICE

Ironically, while the ability to get by on second-rate foods may be essential to human survival in times of famine, it has fed an obsession with junk which threatens the species

I'm not asking you to trust me or have faith, I will be explaining everything to you. I am asking you to keep an open mind and to use your common sense.

If you assumed your weight problem was caused by eating too much of your favorite foods, you probably also assumed that by asking you to change your eating habits I was getting you to give up eating your favorite foods.

Previously I asked you to forget about any preconceptions you had as to your ideal weight. Now I'm asking you to reevaluate what you regard as your favorite foods. In order to remove the brainwashing, I need you to keep your mind open. We need to strip away the misinformation and get back to the facts. When you discover the truth, as I did, you will realize that eating can always be a pleasure and you will never need to worry about having a weight problem again.

Nature intended us to be drawn to the specific foods that are best for us by making them taste the best to us. It also gave us the ability to acquire a taste for second- and third-rate foods, so that we can avoid starvation when our favorite foods are not available. These days we can just go shopping and easily find all our first-rate foods.

> *Nature did not intend us to eat inferior foods if our favorite foods are available. However, this is exactly what we do, and we regard foods that are bad for us as our favorites not as a result of free choice or taste but because of intensive and highly effective brainwashing.*

We have no difficulty in accepting that taste varies from one individual to another. Yet we tend to think of foods as tasting good or bad, even though the next person may think the complete opposite.

The food we eat at home informs and influences our taste buds. Why do Italians love pasta, whereas the British love potatoes and Indians prefer rice?

If you believe the distinction between foods that taste good and foods that taste bad is down to some inherent quality in the foods, why do tastes differ from person to person and why do our own tastes alter during the course of our life? I wouldn't touch blue cheese when I was a child, but as an adult I acquired a taste for it. We can also unacquire tastes.

An unacquired taste

When I was a child, the high point of any birthday party was the cake. We never started with it, we had to eat our sandwiches first and so the cake became the special treat. We were brainwashed by our parents to believe it was the most marvelous thing we could be given to eat.

My excitement was at fever pitch when it was finally brought out. The actual taste doesn't come to mind, but I can remember the thick frosting on the outside and the sticky jam in the layers underneath, and how good it seemed to look on the plate.

I decided I would have an endless supply of it when I was a grown-up. Yet what happened? By the time I could, I no longer had any desire whatsoever to eat birthday cake. The appeal had worn off. Why? Because I was no longer being brainwashed into thinking it was a special treat. I could see it for what it really was.

It was when I started looking more deeply into the principle of acquired taste that I discovered the third important piece of evidence which enabled me to crack the overeating problem. Just as we can acquire a taste for certain foods, we can unacquire it too. In fact, it's the same process. Take tea, for example. Many people start out drinking coffee with sugar. Then one day they decide to cut it out. Unaware of this, you give them a cup with their usual two spoons of sugar and they react almost as if you'd given them poison. You could say they've unacquired the taste for sugar in coffee, or they've acquired the taste for coffee without sugar. The point is their taste has changed.

Give a child a piece of blue cheese and they'll spit it out in disgust. They're heeding a warning light. Yet later in life they may be offered blue cheese again and this time, despite the warning light, they persevere. They keep eating this semi-rotten, curdled dairy product until they acquire the taste. The blue parts of the cheese are simply mold. Normally, we would throw anything else moldy straight into the gabage can. But eating Stilton, Dolcelatte, Gorgonzola, or Danish Blue seems like the grown-up thing to do, a rite of passage.

The junk food conglomerates and the supermarkets are constantly trying to entice you by introducing new products, but they're just repackaging and remarketing the same old junk. It's brainwashing by Big Food that drives us to acquire a taste for foods that are bad for us despite the warning lights. My eighth instruction is:

FREE YOURSELF FROM SLAVERY TO YOUR CURRENT TASTE BUDS

Since you can learn to enjoy the taste of any food, it makes sense to enjoy the taste of the foods that will keep you slim, fit, and healthy. Human beings have done the opposite. Taste can be acquired and unacquired and we've been brainwashed into acquiring a taste for the wrong foods. However, there's a power infinitely more intelligent and sophisticated than even those responsible for this brainwashing, a power that has given us the tools to work out the truth for ourselves.

Try to remember the first time you tried blue cheese, oysters, beer, or coffee. Was there a warning light? Did you need to bypass it to acquire a taste for those foods? Do you see how your own personal tastes can be overridden by brainwashing?

Nature made taste open to suggestion so we could survive when our favorite foods weren't available. But because of the brainwashing, we no longer follow Nature's Guide.

My method removes the brainwashing and once it's gone you'll find it easy to follow Nature. Your natural instincts will come back and your Sensor will help you to know your favorite foods.

If you try to solve your eating problem WITHOUT undoing the brainwashing, you'll be going on a diet and relying on willpower. It will take a mighty effort and you'll fail.

The beauty of my method is that it's easy. All you have to do is understand it and follow the instructions.

We start smoking in the full knowledge that cigarettes contain poison and that sucking toxic fumes into our lungs is unnatural. We don't even get that far with the first few drags, the foul taste in our mouth is enough to prevent us from inhaling and confirms that this is something evil. However, we've been brainwashed to think that smoking is cool and that it must have tremendous advantages as so many people are doing it, and at the same time we've taken a highly addictive drug. So we persevere until we acquire the taste, or at least no longer find it disgusting, and then find we're trapped by the addiction.

It sounds horrific and it is. The same thing happens with our eating habits. Our natural instincts are always there to give us the warning lights, but brainwashing and addiction cloud the picture. We fall into the trap of eating foods that are bad for us and then we feel we can't stop.

HOW WE FOOLED OURSELVES

How were we duped into ignoring Nature's Guide and confusing junk food with the real thing?

Animals found ways to store food so that they could survive in lean times. Our ancestors also knew the importance of food storage and they quickly discovered the drawback with food that gets left uneaten: it goes off. In fact, it gets eaten by other creatures, namely bacteria.

We see bacteria as an enemy, but they're just as much a part of Nature's plan as we are. They just happen to like the same foods as we do. So our ancestors developed ingenious methods for preserving their food, such as cooking, canning, bottling, salting, sweetening, pickling, smoking, and refining. In every case they were effectively making the food inedible to bacteria by removing most of the properties that made it food in the first place, the nutrients. If it's not good enough for bacteria, it's not good enough for us!

It was a way of keeping alive when favorite foods were in short supply. And it worked, sustaining sailors on long voyages for example. But they suffered from being deprived of essential nutrients, developing diseases such as scurvy and rickets, which could only be cured by the fresh fruit and vegetables available on dry land.

Since the 19th century, more and more people have moved from the countryside to towns and cities and access to fresh food for all grew increasingly difficult. Fresh fruit and vegetables became luxuries available only to the wealthy, and so the demand for processed foods began. Fruit tastes so delicious mainly because of its natural sweetness. Humans' taste for fruit existed millions of years before we invented junk food and it's no coincidence that the junk peddled to us by Big Food also tends to be sweet.

Most preprepared food is sweetened in an attempt to replicate the taste of the food designed for us—fruit in its natural state, not cooked to a pulp and made into pies and jams. We also add fruit to bland foods to make them more palatable; apple sauce with pork, or cranberry with turkey. But what happens when the natural sweetness of fresh fruit is not available? The solution our ancestors came up with was one that would cause the biggest single threat to our wellbeing: the addition of refined sugar.

Sugar is added to so many processed foods. This doesn't just include so-called sweet foods. Look on the packaging. It's also added to canned vegetables, baked beans, cereals, yoghurt, and dried meats and is often used as a preservative. As well as mimicking the sweetness of fresh fruit, sugar is also an addictive drug. Even small quantities of sugar in so-called savory processed foods addict us, making us buy them again and again. I will explain more about this in the next chapter.

Processed foods became big business and soon we were all at the mercy of commerce. Today we are utterly dependent on supermarkets which sell us foods we can store at home for months, even years, before eating.

Love kills

When I say that our parents play a big part in the brainwashing, I don't wish to demonize them. While the junk food conglomerates have no concern for the health and wellbeing of their customers, most parents clearly try to do the right thing for their children. The trouble is most of them don't know how.

They encourage their children to eat foods that trigger a warning light and to finish everything on their plate, regardless of how hungry they are. Most parents regard it as their duty to instill these habits in their children, believing it will help them to be strong and healthy.

As I have shown, the opposite is the case. The tragedy is that the people who care most about our health are often those who damage it. Parents who read this book have a marvelous opportunity not only to solve their own eating problems but also to insure that their children do not suffer in later life. Question the brainwashing that you were brought up with and instead apply Nature's Guide.

Nature knows the importance of water for all animals. When food is processed, it loses most of its nutritional value. It also loses its natural water content, which is absolutely vital to us.

As babies we depend on water before we begin to eat solids. Our mother's milk is 88% water and we take in our vital nutrients in liquid form. As we mature, our digestive system continues to prefer foods with a high water content, finding it easier to extract the nutrients and get rid of the waste.

We can survive for weeks or even months without food, but without water we would struggle to survive for more than a few days. By eating the high-water-content foods in Nature's Guide, your favorite foods, you will restore your body's natural balance.

SUMMARY

- **You can acquire a taste for virtually anything.**
- **Fortunately taste can also be unacquired.**
- **Our favorite foods are not an acquired taste.**
- **Free yourself from slavery to your current taste buds and eating habits.**
- **Processing kills the vital nutrients in foods.**
- **Mother's milk is 88% water. Our digestive system continues to prefer foods with a high water content.**

Top Tip No. 12

Keep your Body Balanced

You'll soon be unacquiring your taste for the junk you've been brainwashed to eat. The foods that Nature chose for us are high in water content, just as we are high in water content. A healthy human body is over 60% water and we need to make sure that this vital water content is preserved. Fruit and vegetables are high in water content. Eat them every day. Even foods we don't think of as containing liquid, like bananas, are 75% water.

CHAPTER 13

MEAT AND DAIRY

AN UNNATURAL APPETITE

We rear animals because we regard them as a vital source of food, but we were not designed to eat animals or animal products

The foods we get from animals—meat, dairy and eggs—have been sold to us through an incredibly powerful and prolonged campaign of brainwashing. By meat, I mean the flesh of all animals, fish, and seafood, and by dairy I mean milk and all its by-products. These foods are presented to us as sources of life giving nutrients and as vital for our health and strength.

The traditional Sunday roast is the special meal of the week. We celebrate Christmas or Thanksgiving with a turkey. Easter means a young lamb might be put on the table. And so it goes on. We've developed a tradition of celebrating and rewarding ourselves with meat.

This is strange when you come to think of it, because not only does meat provide us with barely any nutrients at all, it's also virtually tasteless, needs complicated preparation to make it edible, and is extremely difficult to digest. We've been sold the idea that we need meat to make us big and strong, yet you and I know full well that the biggest, strongest animals on the planet eat no meat. Those who tell you that meat is a vital source of protein point not to the vegetarian elephant, rhino, or giraffe but to the carnivorous lion, the King of the Jungle.

But is the lion a role model we should aspire to? OK, it's a powerful beast, but it's nowhere near as strong as the elephant. The lion sleeps 20 hours a day, while the vegetarian giraffe sleeps for a maximum of two hours a day. The orangutan, a creature very similar to humans, also lives on vegetation and swings about energetically for all but six hours every day.

To adopt the eating habits of a carnivore that bears no resemblance to us in either its genetic make-up or lifestyle is ridiculous, especially when there are numerous animals very closely related to us that rely on fruit and vegetables, have boundless energy and strength, and do not suffer from weight problems.

In Chapter 8, we described the Plastic Bag Syndrome and learned we do not need to eat meat for protein. The body produces protein itself, provided we are getting our 20 necessary amino acids. Amino acids fall into two groups, essential and nonessential. Eleven of the amino acids, those called nonessential, are already in our system. The nine essential amino acids need to be sourced externally, therefore through our intake. These essential amino acids are found in plants and best replenished by eating vegetables. We do not need animals or animal products to get protein.

We were not designed to eat meat. In fact, it's hard to imagine a food less suitable for human consumption.

MAN AND MEAT

Carnivores of all sizes have long, powerful fangs and razor-sharp incisors, as well as sharp, powerful claws for gripping and tearing flesh. Compare your teeth and fingernails to the teeth and claws of even a domestic cat—do you really think you have what it takes to kill and dissect an animal with your bare hands and teeth? If you tried—and I'm not suggesting you do—you would have considerable difficulty consuming it. Apart from the unpleasantness of having to drink another animal's blood, it's extremely difficult to chew. If you did manage to force some down your throat, your digestive system would not thank you for it. Of all the foods people eat, meat is the most difficult to digest and dispose of. The stomach of a carnivore contains much more hydrochloric acid than the human stomach. This is what enables it to break meat down efficiently, and its relatively short intestines enable it to dispose of the waste quickly. Humans are not physically cut out to eat meat.

Meat has a high fat content and a relatively low water content, and cooking it lowers the water content further. Our stomachs are designed to digest food with a low fat and high water content. Meat also has a very high protein content and we do not have the enzymes necessary to digest large quantities of concentrated fat and protein efficiently. The putrefying waste takes about 20 hours to pass through our long intestines, and there will be traces of meat in your digestive tract weeks after eating it. Eating meat obstructs the natural elimination cycle. As your body struggles and fails to break down the flesh, your system builds up a backlog of undigested matter which then turns into fat.

If you could see inside your body, you would appreciate the damage that meat does to your insides. It's not just your stomach that suffers. Your kidneys can't flush it all out of your system, and all your other organs work overtime in an attempt to rectify the situation. But your body is incredibly resilient and the mere fact that you're still alive seems like evidence that there's nothing too horrendous going on inside. Think again. Just because your body has coped up until now, is that really a sensible argument for continuing to treat it like a waste disposal unit? You're reading this book because you have a weight problem. Follow my method and your body will be getting all the nutrients it needs from the right foods and you will not only be your ideal weight, you will also take more pleasure in eating and be bursting with energy and vitality.

NEITHER THE STOMACH NOR THE HEART

Food we think of as fresh is often processed. When I was a boy chicken was a luxury. Today, thanks to a string of bad news stories concerning red meat, chicken is the main meat staple. It's cheap and has not yet been blamed for any chronic degenerative diseases. But if you saw the way battery hens are reared and pumped with hormones, I doubt you'd ever be able to get excited about your roast chicken again.

These days animals are not so much reared as processed. We don't go and see their appalling conditions ourselves and we block our minds to the hideous methods of mass production. We're hoodwinked by friendly images and tempting words from the meat industry. We're told these foods are of genuine nutritional benefit and we're led to believe we need them to be strong and healthy. Who are we to question it? We've been sold the same line from infancy, even by our own parents, who were sold it by their parents.

> *"Place a small child in a crib with a rabbit and an apple. If it eats the rabbit and plays with the apple, I'll buy you a new car."*
> Harvey Diamond, co-author *Fit For Life*

We aren't emotionally designed to eat meat either. When you're in the countryside on a glorious spring day and you see new-born lambs frolicking in the lush, green pastures, do you begin to salivate and want to rush into the field to pounce on one, tear its throat out, and feast on the blood and gore as a wolf would? Or do you think, "Aren't they cute?"

Compare your behavior to that of a true carnivore. Even domesticated dogs have to be restrained when faced with a field of lambs. You might argue that as humans we have become civilized in a way a dog has not and, therefore, we know better than to commit such "animalistic" acts. But the irony is that those lambs are being bred and nurtured solely so that we can kill and eat them.

A whole industry has been created so that we can eat meat without having to kill it ourselves, or even think about the mass slaughter. In the endless quest for cost-efficiency and bigger profits, Big Food has come to treat animals with staggering cruelty. The tiny cages in which they're permanently confined bear absolutely no resemblance to their natural habitat. For an idea of a battery hen's life, imagine having to spend every day in a wire cage the size of a bathtub with four other people. When we're presented with images of such horror, we react with revulsion and pity.

Even the language we use severs the connection between the meat and the animal it comes from. Why do you think we talk of pork, beef, veal, and venison rather than pig, cow, calf, and deer? It's much easier to tuck into a portion of meat if we don't have to think about the living animal.

Let me make it clear, I'm not presenting the moral arguments against eating meat. I'm not appealing to your conscience, I'm just showing you that humans are not natural carnivores. We lack the physical attributes and we lack the instinct.

It's in our nature to love animals. We keep dogs, cats, hamsters, rabbits, guinea pigs, gerbils, turtles, fish, even rats and snakes, not for eating but for companionship. We spend a lot of money on them. We love to play with them, watch them, talk to them, and feed them. We take them to the vet when they're sick, and when they die, we make graves for them and grieve. Can you think of any other carnivore that chooses to co-habit with other species the way we do, without ever thinking of eating them?

I know several people who have reared chickens and pigs with the intention of eating them, but when it came to the kill they couldn't bring themselves to do it and ended up keeping them as pets.

THE DAIRY DELUSION

The favorite food of all new-born mammals is their mother's milk. It provides all the vitamins and nutrients they need and we don't question that. We make no attempt to vary its intake or complement it with vitamin supplements. We recognize the baby is getting the exact food Nature designed for it.

When we see any animal suckling on its mother's breast, be it a calf, lamb, kitten or puppy, we instinctively have a feeling of wellbeing. If milk is the natural food that contains all the nutrients we need, surely it makes sense to drink as much of it as we can throughout our lives?

When I was a child, milk was a staple in our household. Delivered every day by the milkman, it was given to me cold on my return from school and warm with a spot of honey if I was feeling unwell or finding it difficult to sleep. It was sold to me as the elixir of life. I initially found this aspect of the brainwashing tricky to overcome. It's only recently that the true damage caused by consuming dairy products has come to light. It causes heart disease and diabetes and aggravates eczema, hay fever, asthma, and osteoporosis.

Remember, the baby is getting the exact food designed for that baby. The milk of all mammals is specially formulated with the specific balance of vitamins, iron, calcium, and other nutrients that the specific infant requires. You wouldn't give a new-born baby cows' milk. The milk of each mammal is unique.

Milk is designed only for babies. Can you think of any other animals that continue drinking milk in adulthood, other than humans and their pets? I can't. Not even cows! Furthermore, we don't even continue drinking our own milk, we switch to that of another species!

Dairy may be easier to consume than meat, but it's also very difficult to digest. This is because of lactose, a substance in all milk products. Lactase, the enzyme which can digest lactose, occurs in the human body when we're babies in order to digest our mother's milk. It leaves our bodies as we grow. This clearly demonstrates that we're not designed to consume dairy products as adults. Rennet enzymes, extracted from mammals' stomachs, are used in the production of most cheeses to coagulate the milk. When we eat cheese, we're usually also eating a meat product.

> ### Babar
> In the illustrated children's book, The Story of Babar, *the animals are humanized, not only by giving them clothes, houses, and cars but also by making them susceptible to human error. Babar becomes King of the Elephants when the previous king dies from eating a poisonous mushroom. Wild animals choose their food using their Sensor. A real elephant would have been able to tell the mushroom was fatal. Unlike us, wild animals are still guided by their instincts and still follow Nature's Guide.*

WHAT ARE OUR FAVORITE FOODS?

It's clear that adults were not designed to consume any dairy products including milk, particularly not the milk of another species. While mother's milk is the stuff of life for infant mammals, it's clearly not designed for after infancy. It's also clear that both physically and emotionally humans were not designed to eat meat. To ignore these points is to go against Nature's plan.

So what does that leave? Fruit, vegetables, nuts, and grains. I can hear the cries of anguish. "Does that mean I'll have to become a vegan?" No.

Vegans do not eat meat or animal products. Remember with my method there are no restrictions. If you can't contemplate a life without meat, fish, or dairy, you don't have to. Remember the Junk Margin.

Like most people, I used to find the thought of becoming a vegan weird. It ceased to bother me once I'd discovered the secret to my weight problem. I realized there was nothing to be afraid of. I was making no sacrifice whatsoever and my food intake could remain as varied as I liked. I also realized that fresh fruit, nuts, vegetables, and grains formed the main part of most people's intake anyway.

Think of a typical everyday meal: lamb, rice, carrots, peas and salad. The meat is only a small proportion and in any case, there's a huge variety of fruits, nuts, vegetables, and grains to choose from.

There's an almost limitless selection of first-rate foods in the stores these days and with my method your taste buds and hunger will always be satisfied by your favorite foods, so you won't feel deprived and you'll be your ideal weight.

SUMMARY

- We are not physically designed to eat meat.
- We are not emotionally designed to eat meat.
- Mother's milk is the only milk suitable for us, and only during infancy.
- To eat meat and dairy products to get protein and calcium is to fall for the Plastic Bag Syndrome.
- Reducing the meat and dairy content of your intake will not take away the variety.

Top Tip No.13

Eat with your Heart

There are certain things that we're not emotionally equipped to eat. A true carnivore doesn't feel sentimental towards animals. Follow your heart.

CHAPTER 14

OUR FAVORITE FOODS

IN THIS CHAPTER
• *WHAT OUR CLOSEST RELATIVES CAN TEACH US*
• *THE ABUNDANCE OF NATURAL FOODS* • *COOKING*
• *THE NINTH INSTRUCTION* • *WHY ARE YOU ALWAYS HUNGRY?*

THE NATURAL CHOICE

I've explained why certain foods are not designed for us. Now let's see which ones are

It's time to establish exactly which foods were designed for human consumption. In order to do so, it helps to look back at humans before they began to tamper with food, before they discovered the secret of fire and started cooking, planting crops, or rearing livestock. A good way to do this is to look at the animals that most closely resemble us.

The great apes are our closest relatives, in particular the chimpanzee, which shares 99% of our DNA. Like us, chimps are omnivores, they eat fruit, vegetation, and meat. Their favorite food by far is fruit, followed by leaves. They eat around 60% fruit and 20% leaves. Seeds and blossoms account for around 10%, and only about 5% is meat and insects.

Given the choice, a chimpanzee would much rather eat fruit

and leaves. Does that make the chimpanzee's life repetitive and dull? Not a bit of it. A chimp will find pleasure in as many as 300 different types of plant. You may think you enjoy a varied intake, but when was the last time you put 300 different food items in your shopping basket?

NATURE'S VARIETY SHOW

A quick look around my local supermarket revealed the abundance of natural foods which can be eaten raw; see the table opposite. It's by no means a comprehensive list.

Fruit ticks all the boxes in Nature's Guide. It looks good, smells good, and tastes good. So much so that humans have learned to extract the flavor from fruit and add it to other things. We give taste to most desserts, cakes, and confectionery by adding fresh fruit or fruit essences.

If meat tastes good in itself, why the need to cook it and add seasoning, sauces, and condiments? Have you ever felt an apple could do with a pinch of salt? Does your banana taste better if you add pepper? Of course not. Fruit requires no added flavoring. On the contrary, we add fruit and vegetables to bland foods like meat to give them flavor: apple sauce with pork, cranberry sauce with turkey, garlic and mustard with beef, paprika and onion with chicken, etc.

When it comes to flavoring drinks, we also turn to fruit: blackberry, orange, lemon, lime, strawberry, raspberry, peach, pineapple, banana. And not just soft drinks either. In addition to the grapes and hops that go into wine and beer, we flavor spirits

FRUIT	VEGETABLES	SEEDS, NUTS AND HERBS
Apples	Lettuce	Almonds
Pears	Arugula	Brazil Nuts
Peaches	Spinach	Cashews
Bananas	Asparagus	Coconuts
Pineapples	Cabbage	Macadamia Nuts
Plums	Carrot	Pecans
Oranges	Celery	Peanuts
Grapes	Peas	Pistachios
Lemons	Radishes	Walnuts
Satsumas	Pepper	Chestnuts
Clementines	Onion	Hazelnuts
Tangerines	Scallions	Sesame Seeds
Mandarins	Beans	Sunflower Seeds
Melons	Bean Sprouts	Caraway Seeds
Mangos	Chicory	Poppy Seeds
Apricots	Cauliflower	Pumpkin Seeds
Cherries	Snow Peas	Oregano
Kiwis	Broccoli	Parsley
Pomegranates	Pak Choi	Rosemary
Strawberries	Fennel	Tarragon
Raspberries	Sprouts	Thyme
Blackberries	Cucumber	Basil
Loganberries	Beets	Coriander
Gooseberries	Celeriac	
Redcurrants	Chard	
Blackcurrants	Garlic	
Tomatoes	Mushrooms	
Avocados	Leeks	

with orange, lemon, cherry, apricot, juniper, sloe, and more. The blurb on wine bottle labels often boasts something like "bursting with the flavor of summer fruits, a combination of rich raspberry, blackberry and cherry." Nowadays, there are even fruit-flavored beers.

Fruit appeals to our natural instincts more than any other food. This is not simply a question of taste. Taste is closely associated with hunger, and hunger is your body's way of telling you that it needs certain nutrients. Fruit provides those nutrients.

Earlier we discussed the importance of high-water-content foods to aid digestion, the absorption of nutrients, and the disposal of wastes. Fruit is your digestive system's best friend. It requires barely any breaking down and passes very quickly from the stomach to the intestines, where the goodness is easily extracted. It aids the natural elimination cycle and the waste is easily disposed of, avoiding the build-up of indigestible matter that turns into fat.

Water is the most vital nutrient for humans. The human body is 70% water. It lubricates our body. If you become dehydrated, your system cannot function properly. Fruit consists mainly of water, some as much as 90%. Fruit is the food that naturally provides us with the water we need.

In fact, the more you look at the design of fruit, the more you realize how ingenious it is. Whether it's a banana, which comes in its own natural, easy-to-remove wrapper, or an apple that stays firm and shiny for weeks, always ready to eat, the Earth is brimming with an abundance of fruit, provided for us in attractive and convenient packages and offering a vast variety of delicious flavors.

Fruit remains cool and refreshing even on hot days. It satisfies both our hunger and our thirst. It's packed full of the minerals and vitamins we need to be healthy and strong. There's very little waste when we digest fruit, and we easily dispose of the little there is, which means that, in contrast to meat, it gives you the energy and vitality essential for enjoying life. You can't have too much energy. Energy is the source of human happiness. The more you have, the better you feel. It's cool to eat fruit, and fruit's cool to eat.

We can learn a lot about our natural instincts by observing the behavior of infants. Observe babies' eating habits before the brainwashing kicks in. They begin life wanting only their mother's milk. When the time comes to move on to solids, the food they will eat most readily is fruit.

COOKING

Fresh fruit, fresh vegetables, nuts, and seeds (nuts are essentially a type of seed) are clearly the ideal foods for humans. These foods provide us with all the nutrients we require and can be eaten in their natural state.

We have been cooking food ever since we learned how to use fire around 800,000 years ago in the Stone Age, so long that our bodies have evolved and adapted to be able to deal without problems with a limited intake of cooked food. This means that it's fine to eat foods that grow naturally but cannot be eaten raw, such as most root vegetables, wholegrains, and pulses, as our bodies can digest these and assimilate the nutrients without much difficulty.

WHOLEGRAINS	VEGETABLES AND PULSES
Rice	Most Root Vegetables
Flour: Rye/Wheat/Corn	Artichoke
Barley	Olives
Cous-Cous	Seaweed
Breads and Crackers	Corn-on-the-cob
Pasta	Eggplant
Millet	Dried Beans
Polenta	Lentils
Cracked Wheat	Chickpeas
Cereals	Split and Black-Eyed Peas

These foods are not first-rate like fruit, but they are not nearly so bad for you as meat, dairy, and other junk, and can be included in your intake without unduly clogging up your system. If you are cooking anything, try to cook it in the simplest and lightest way possible as this will minimize the loss of nutrients and you will still satisfy your hunger.

Stone Age humans may have discovered fire, but their intake still consisted mainly of raw foraged foods such as roots, shoots, nuts, berries, and seeds.

Vegetable oils can also be digested without problem, even though they are processed. It's best to stick to oils that have been extracted using cold pressing because when the oil is heated the properties of the oil molecules and unsaturated fatty acids change, destroying their nutritional value and making them toxic. For the same reason it's best not to cook in oil.

WHY AM I HAVING TO TELL YOU THIS?

The evidence against junk is indisputable, so it's hard to understand how such an intelligent species as human beings has allowed itself to consume so much of it.

Why are the billboards not showing us images of fresh fruit? Why isn't children's television punctuated with ads for fresh vegetables?

Big Food doesn't make its profits by selling foods in their natural state. That's a small part of the market. The real money lies in tampering with natural foods, processing them beyond recognition, then presenting them in new ways, and making consumers believe they're getting added value, when all they're really getting is the same old junk and a weight problem.

To make matters worse, the so-called experts to whom we look for guidance keep changing their minds about which foods are good for us and which are bad, and send out such mixed messages that the result is confusion.

Even when they do get it right, they fail to go all the way. The warnings about red meat and full-fat milk were long overdue, but what do they recommend instead? Chicken and skimmed milk. Why? Either meat and milk are good for us or they're not.

I asked you to keep an open mind so that you can overcome the brainwashing and confusion. If you think for yourself and use your own common sense, it's easy to see the reality. Humans and their ancestors have been on Earth for millions of years. The mass production of processed foods has only taken place over the last 200 years. We have thrived by eating food in its natural state.

My ninth instruction is: ***BEWARE OF PROCESSED FOODS***

A FRUITLESS EXERCISE

We have come to accept processed food as a normal part of life and this brainwashing needs to be reversed. Our natural instincts have worked for millions of years and the good news is they're still there. You just need to learn to listen to them again.

Processing strips food of its vital nutrients, including its natural water content. You might think that cooking it in water or stock, or adding water later, or drinking with the meal will compensate. Buying yourself a pack of powdered tomato soup to have at the office may be convenient since all you have to do is add hot water, but this concoction bears no relation to fresh tomatoes. Adding liquid back doesn't restore the natural water content or the nutrients. That's not how our digestive system works; it's the Plastic Bag Syndrome.

Your digestive system ingeniously extracts the nutrients from the food you eat, distributes them to the correct parts of your body, and disposes of the waste. It's a highly sophisticated machine, but it was only designed to perform efficiently with the right fuel. Eat food not designed for it and it won't be able to dispose of the waste as Nature intended. Instead it will store it where it can, and that's where the unsightly bulges appear.

Processed food has had its high water content removed and is therefore difficult to digest, and drinking during the meal can make the problem worse by diluting the digestive juices in your stomach.

When our stomach sends the message that we're hungry, we naturally interpret it as the need for food. It's not quite so simple. The message is actually calling for specific nutrients and it's up to us to provide the foods that contain those nutrients.

We have seen that food only tastes good when you're hungry. So why do some people continue to eat when they've stuffed themselves? With all that food inside them, surely they can't still be hungry. And yet they still have the desire to eat.

THE REASON IS THEY <u>ARE</u> STILL HUNGRY

Hunger is the body asking for nutrients. If the food you eat doesn't supply those nutrients, it will continue to demand them, despite being bloated.

This is the key to my method and to solving your weight problem. Understand why overeating is the direct result of eating the wrong foods, and the door to your prison will swing open.

The digestive process can be an extremely energy-sapping exercise if you eat the wrong foods. We tend not to be aware of this because it goes on quietly inside us. Have you ever wondered why we often fall asleep after Christmas lunch? For the same reason that lions and other carnivores spend so much of their lives asleep.

Fruit leaves us bounding with energy because it's so easy to digest and full of nutrients. Junk is hard and slow to break down, very low in nutrients, and clogs up the whole digestive process. Every cell suffers when it's deprived of the right nutrients, leaving you permanently tired.

Junk leaves you hungry and if you try to satisfy that hunger by eating more junk, the problem just gets worse. It's this vicious circle that leads to people becoming grossly overweight.

A large glass of water is usually enough to quench your thirst. Water contains all the nutrients your body is asking for when it sends the message that you're thirsty. You know when your thirst is quenched and you don't need any more water. But try quenching your thirst with beer or processed soft drinks. You can drink two or three and still want more. Alcohol and the junk in processed soft drinks cause dehydration—the very opposite of what you are trying to achieve—and so you continue to feel thirsty. The same principle applies to hunger and eating. Unless you provide your body with the nutrients it needs, it will continue to send the message that you're hungry. My tenth instruction is:

SATISFY YOUR HUNGER WITH YOUR FAVORITE FOODS

Let me make it clear, I'm not telling you what you can and can't eat. Remember, the Junk Margin. But your hunger can only be satisfied with your favorite foods. You'll enjoy the delicious flavors of natural food at every meal; you'll be bursting with energy; you'll be slim, fit, and healthy; and you'll find that junk quickly loses its appeal.

SUMMARY

- Fruit looks good, smells good, tastes good, is the easiest food to digest, and gives us boundless energy. It's clearly our favorite food.
- Processing food kills nutrients, adds toxins, and removes water.
- Overeating is the result of eating the wrong foods which do not satisfy your hunger.
- Satisfy your hunger with natural foods.

Top Tip No.14

Cooking

When you're cooking, keep it quick and simple. Cooking destroys nutrients and overcooking can turn your favorite foods into junk. You will be more relaxed as you find your favorite foods can be simply and quickly prepared and you don't have to spend hours in the kitchen.

CHAPTER 15

SUGAR ADDICTION

IN THIS CHAPTER
• OBSESSED WITH SUGAR
*• HOW THE ADDICTION WORKS • THE ILLUSION OF
PLEASURE • CHOCAHOLISM • SUGAR SUBSTITUTES • SALT*

SWEET AND SOUR

We view drug addiction with horror. The irony is, most of us are consuming large quantities of an addictive drug without even being aware of it—SUGAR

When I refer to sugar here, I mean processed or refined sugar artificially extracted from food, not the natural sugar in such foods as fruit. Natural fruit sugar causes the body no problems at all. On the contrary, it's a fantastic source of energy. Human beings designed processed sugar in an attempt to mimic the sweet taste of our favorite foods. It's not the calories in the sugar that are the real problem: It's the way the substance reacts once inside the body and clogs up the digestive system. Even small amounts of sugar undermine the efficiency of our metabolism and cause weight gain. It's one of the most dangerous forms of junk for your health and wellbeing, and it's addictive.

> **The myth of the instant hit**
>
> *There can be a tendency to eat a chocolate bar, cookies, or other confectionery as a quick fix between meals to keep going. This can cause what's often referred to as a "sugar rush" or "instant hit." This may sound like a positive thing, but it isn't. While the release of the natural energy in fruit is controlled by the digestive system, the sudden introduction of processed sugar has a disastrous effect on your blood sugar level, artificially increasing it, which makes you feel nervous and on edge, and then causing it to crash. As your blood sugar level subsequently drops, you feel low and lethargic and as processed sugar contains no nutrients, the feelings of tiredness and demotivation are increased. You probably won't realise how lethargic you've become until you follow my method and rediscover your natural energy levels.*

HOW WE BECOME ADDICTED

As processed sugar leaves your blood stream, it causes an empty, restless, out-of-sorts feeling. This is withdrawal. If you consume more sugar at this point, it temporarily relieves this feeling, creating the illusion that the sugar has made you happy. In fact, all it has done is taken you from feeling low to feeling okay. But you were okay before you took the first dose of sugar. You weren't missing anything. Once withdrawal starts, you feel the need for it again and again just to get you back to the level you were on before the first dose.

In fact you never quite get back to where you were before you started because your body builds up a tolerance, so every time you take it, you need more to get the same relief, and every time it leaves your system, you sink lower. The longer you go on trying to relieve the withdrawal by consuming more sugar, the lower your wellbeing sinks and the more you feel you need it.

Below is a graph illustrating a processed sugar addict's level of wellbeing as he goes through life.

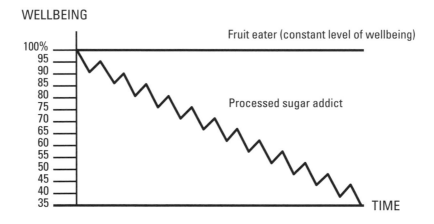

There are genuine highs and lows and stresses and strains in life, but for the purposes of this exercise and for the sake of clarity, we're going to ignore those and focus exclusively on the effect that sugar addiction has on your level of wellbeing over time. We're going to assume that before you get hooked, you're on 100%. Being on a high means having no problems.

As an addict, you're permanently below 100%, i.e. below the level of wellbeing you would have had if you were not an addict, because you're constantly withdrawing, but you're not aware of it because it's so slight and you regard that state as normal. This is why eating cakes, chocolates, and candy makes you feel below par. Assume you're ten points below because of the withdrawal and you recover five of those points when you consume more processed sugar. You receive a little boost, but you're still below the level you would be at if you weren't an addict in the first place. Perhaps you're thinking, "So what? Won't that five-point gain make me feel better, even if it's an illusion?" Would you put on tight shoes just for the relief of removing them? This is what all drug addicts effectively do, but only because they don't understand the trap they're in. As time passes and you go through life as a sugar addict, you slide further and further down as your wellbeing declines both physically and mentally.

At first it doesn't bother us, but as you go deeper and deeper into the pit, the situation continues to deteriorate. You become fat, lethargic, and depressed. Your wellbeing level is therefore gradually but continuously declining and the level you come back to when you consume processed sugar goes down in proportion.

If we woke up one morning twice the size we were when we went to bed and ten times more lethargic, we'd be shocked. But because this is a gradual process, we're scarcely even aware of it. The physical withdrawal from processed sugar causes no pain, is very slight, and passes quickly. The deprivation you feel when you want, say, a chocolate bar but can't have one is entirely mental and caused by the illusion that you're being forced to do without a genuine pleasure or crutch. Once the brainwashing has been removed and you can see processed sugar for what it really is, you will no longer suffer this feeling of deprivation.

The great news is that when you start eating your favorite foods, you can return to the level of wellbeing you would have had all your life if you had never become addicted in the first place. The physical withdrawal from processed sugar is easy to deal with and disappears very quickly; the body starts to recover immediately, and, provided you no longer see processed sugar as any sort of pleasure or crutch, you won't feel you're making any sacrifice and **YOU WILL BE FREE**.

EVERY OVEREATER WISHES THEY COULD STOP

The beautiful truth is they can, provided they understand the trap they're in and follow my instructions. You now understand that overeating is caused by consuming the wrong foods. When you eat the right foods your Sensor, Gauge, and digestive system all work as they should and the nutrients satisfy your hunger. Processed sugar is not one of our favorite foods. It causes overeating, not only because it won't satisfy your hunger but also because it's an addictive substance and you will eat more and more in an attempt to fill the void you feel as it leaves your body. However, the drug does not fill the void, it creates it.

As with all addictive drugs, it's not the physical withdrawal from the processed sugar which keeps you hooked but the brainwashing that goes with it.

From an early age we're led to believe that there's something special about sweet foods: "If you finish your main course, you can have a dessert." Of course we're going to regard the dessert as a special treat. The illusion continues as we grow up and is reinforced by everybody around us who have themselves been brainwashed into believing that a cake or a box of chocolates brings happiness, when it really brings a feeling of emptiness, a craving for more, and a weight problem.

We're taught that the highlight of a celebration is the cake. Once you understand that it's the company and the event that are enjoyable, not the sugary foods, you'll find that you can go to parties and other functions and still have a great time without touching the cakes, biscuits, and desserts and without feeling in the slightest deprived. On the contrary, you'll be able to rejoice in the fact that you don't have to shovel that mass of indigestible, fat-triggering junk into your body.

Chocaholics

Have you ever opened a box of chocolates on your own with the intention of eating only one, and found that before you know it you've scoffed the lot? Why do we do it? There's no pleasure in it. Physically you feel bloated and sick, while emotionally you feel disgusted with yourself, miserable, and out of control.

The first chocolate leaves you feeling unsatisfied, so you think, "Just one more." Again, it fails to satisfy, so you keep going, until before you know it, you've eaten the entire box, including the ones you don't like!

Most chocolate is made from three basic ingredients: cocoa, which contains an addictive drug similar to caffeine called theobromine; processed sugar; and cow's milk, which is intended for calves. Although it's true that some chocolate is more processed and contains more junk than others, there's no such thing as "pure" chocolate. It's all processed and it all contains theobromine.

The chocolate box scenario is typical of addictive behavior. Addicts often feed their addiction in private, as they don't want to admit to it. They see it as shameful and often lie to cover it up.

The natural sugar in unprocessed foods such as fruit is easily digested and like all other nutrients travels through the body and feeds it. In its natural form, it's the primary fuel for your mind. When you eat fruit, the natural sugar, fructose, enters your body combined with fiber and water. These act together to create the glucose necessary for your brain to function. This process results in a gradual release of energy. Processed sugar is a poison. Insulin is the hormone which regulates glucose in your body. Processed sugar triggers an excess of insulin in the stomach which overrides your digestive system, making it incapable of breaking down the other foods which then turn into fat.

MANUFACTURED

The process of refining, or processing, sugar is very similar to the way the coca plant is processed into cocaine, and poppy seeds processed into heroin. The processing strips away the fiber, vitamins, and minerals from the natural source, leaving behind a crystalline substance that is very sweet and soluble. Processed sugar is extracted from all sorts of food and you will find it called many things.

So beware of barley malt, beet sugar, brown rice syrup, cane juice, corn syrup, dextrose, sucrose, and maple sugar. It's all manufactured and it's all addictive junk.

Perhaps you don't think you have a sugar problem. I suggest you check the labels on every item of food you buy. You may be surprised by the number that contain processed sugar, even preprepared, savory dishes that you don't associate with sweetness, such as soups, bread, pizzas, and potato chips. Fresh fruit and vegetables don't need an ingredients label. They're pure foods in their natural state and the sugar in them does not cause the sudden and extreme fluctuations in blood sugar levels which result in withdrawal and addiction.

Carbohydrates can be an excellent source of energy and you can get them from all sorts of foods: fruits, vegetables, pulses, and wholegrains. These natural carbohydrates are easily digested and turned into energy. However, when grains are processed to make foods such as white bread, white rice, white pasta, and white flour, they can have a similar effect on you as processed sugar. The processing of these carbohydrates removes the rusk, taking away the fiber and nutrients—all the good parts our bodies can use—and the remaining carbohydrate acts like processed sugar and excess insulin is released in your body.

HONEY AND OTHER SWEETENERS

We are predisposed to like sweetness for a good reason: fruit—sweet, delicious fruit, our favorite food. Don't substitute the natural goodness of fruit with processed sugar or alternative sweeteners. Honey is a concentrated food with a low water content. Although it's the favorite food for bees, it's not suitable for us and, like processed sugar, triggers excess insulin in our bodies. Sweeteners are sold as a calorie-free alternative. Leptin is a hormone that helps to regulate your appetite and helps your body to metabolize. Aspartame and other sweeteners are acids which reduce the leptin in your body by as much as 35%. This has a disastrous effect on your ability to gauge your hunger and on your body's ability to metabolize efficiently. Don't confuse powdered fructose, sometimes marketed as "fruit sugar," with the natural fructose in fruit. Once removed from the fruit, it acts exactly like processed sugar. It's junk now that it has been separated from the water, fiber, and other nutrients in natural food. In this form it's simply another additive.

Remember liquids contain processed sugar or sweeteners too: alcohol, fizzy drinks, cordials, and processed juices. There is one drink that contains no sugar at all and is the best thirst quencher on Earth. It's the drink we reach for ahead of any other when we're completely parched: water. Cool, refreshing, oxygen-packed water.

SALT

Natural salt is an essential nutrient and, like sugar, there's enough in your favorite foods: fruits and vegetables. The natural salt in these foods is combined with other organic molecules and this means that our system absorbs it slowly and efficiently without any problems. However, processed or refined salt causes almost as many problems as processed or refined sugar. In large quantities it can even be lethal. In China, a traditional method of suicide was drinking water saturated with salt. One ounce of processed salt causes the body to retain six pounds of excess fluid. When I refer to salt here, I'm referring to processed salt.

Frequently eating foods with added salt has a dangerous effect on several aspects of your health. It increases blood pressure, a major risk factor in heart disease and premature death, and can cause kidney failure, diabetes, osteoporosis, and cancer. This is because processed or refined salt is unbuffered and moves too quickly through the stomach lining causing a surplus in the bloodstream and taking the fluid from our cells to deal with the excess. When a surplus of salt enters the bloodstream, the body is forced to store the salt between the cells until the kidneys can filter it. This causes a caustic, burning effect on the surrounding tissue. For protection, the cells release water into the intercellular fluid to dilute the excess salt. As the cells give up their water, they lose elasticity and shrink. This, in turn, causes an imbalance of the cells' chemistry through a loss of potassium. This disruption of the body's fluid balance scars your muscles and organs.

If you're trying to lose weight or trim down, salt is counter-productive, because it hinders the correct functioning of the body and causes water retention and swelling. Virtually all processed food contains salt. Big Food has discovered that adding salt to food not only increases its shelf life but also makes you carry on eating it because, like processed sugar, it's addictive. We all know that once we start on the salty potato chips or nibbles, there's no hope of stopping until we've scoffed all of them. Avoid having that first one, and there's no problem. We've been brainwashed to think salt brings out the taste in food, but actually it makes it all taste the same—of salt. Food is much more exciting when you can taste its real flavor. If you do use salt, use natural sea salt rather than table salt, because it's not as processed.

SUMMARY

- Processed sugar is addictive, and it's added to almost all junk.
- Addictive drugs do not satisfy the craving, they cause it.
- Processed sugar provides no benefits and creates fat.
- Avoid sugar substitutes.
- Avoid drinks containing processed sugar or sugar substitutes —they're all junk.
- Avoid adding salt to food and enjoy the natural flavors.

Top Tip No. 15

Sweet Foods You Find in Nature

Empty the house of sweet junk and replace it with a bowl of beautiful, fresh fruit. Keep the bowl topped up with your favorite, fresh, juicy fruits. You and your family will be getting all the goodness you need and none of the guilt.

CHAPTER 16

REVERSING THE BRAINWASHING

DISPELLING DELUSIONS

Let's reverse the brainwashing and start seeing foods as they really are

Look closely. What do you think this says?

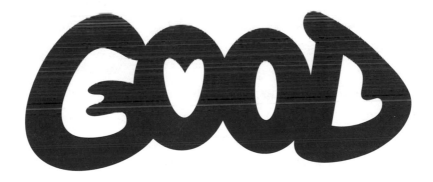

Now hold the book further away. Some people see the word "evil" to begin with, but then see the word "good." Sometimes it's the other way around. Whichever way you see it first, once you're aware of both words, you can no longer convince yourself that there's only one.

Can you see how easy it is to see the same thing in the opposite way when you're given a different perspective?

Since we can be fooled into seeing junk as desirable, it's easy to reverse the process and see it as it really is. It's also easy to see the beauty of natural foods.

A TWO-PRONGED ATTACK

Reversing the brainwashing is surprisingly simple, provided you approach the process with an open mind and do two things. First, take the time to concentrate on the foods intended for you by Nature and start seeing them for what they are: delicious, energy-packed sources of all the nutrients you need to be slim, fit, and healthy. Cut open a ripe, colourful, juicy peach, orange, pineapple or pear; breathe in the amazing aroma; relish the delicious flavor in your mouth; feel the cool, fresh juice; and appreciate the energy and nutrients that your body is going to benefit from with barely any effort. Try new fruits. There are countless varieties available—maybe you've never eaten a mango or a kiwi fruit. Also consider the vast array of fresh, delicious, nutrient-packed, high-water-content vegetables on offer. You can take your pick of carrots, peppers, cabbage, lettuce, radishes, cauliflower, broccoli, tomatoes, avocados, mushrooms, asparagus, and spinach, to name just a few. Like fruit, you can enjoy these raw and in no time create delicious, nourishing dishes. With my method your choice of foods will expand, not reduce.

Second, take the time to see junk for what it really is. Digesting meat takes an average of three days. We are not designed to eat meat. Take a look below to see how ill-equipped we are to consume other animals and how well-equipped to consume our favorite foods.

Meat-eaters: sharp front teeth for tearing, no flat molar teeth for grinding
Herbivores: no sharp front teeth, flat rear molars for grinding
Humans: no sharp front teeth, flat rear molars for grinding

Meat-eaters: intestinal tract is only three times their body length so rapidly decaying meat can pass through quickly
Herbivores: intestinal tract 10–12 times their body length
Humans: intestinal tract 10–12 times their body length

Meat-eaters: strong hydrochloric acid in stomach to digest meat
Herbivores: stomach acid that is 20 times weaker than that of a meat-eater
Humans: stomach acid that is 20 times weaker than that of a meat-eater

Meat-eaters: salivary glands in mouth not developed to predigest grains and fruits
Herbivores: well-developed salivary glands necessary to predigest grains and fruits
Humans: well-developed salivary glands necessary to predigest grains and fruits

Meat-eaters: acid saliva with no enzyme ptyalin to predigest grains
Herbivores: alkaline saliva with ptyalin to predigest grains
Humans: alkaline saliva with ptyalin to predigest grains

Meat-eaters: claws to kill and eat prey
Herbivores: no claws
Humans: no claws

Meat-eaters: no skin pores, perspire through tongue
Herbivores: perspire through skin pores
Humans: perspire through skin pores

If you eat meat think about it while it's in your mouth and try to ascertain exactly what you enjoy. Do you really want to chew this flavourless, dead flesh which will sit in your stomach for ages while your body works overtime trying to digest it and dispose of all the toxins and waste matter and which makes you overweight?

> **••• FACT BOX •••**
> Vegetarians are slimmer, healthier, and closer to
> their ideal weight than nonvegetarians.

Despite the stark contrast between the genuine enjoyment from eating our naturally favorite foods and eating junk, you may still fear that you are going to feel deprived. Smokers who try to quit by using willpower experience a similar fear. They worry that they'll never be able to enjoy a social occasion or handle stress without cigarettes. This is because they don't understand the nicotine trap. People with eating problems make the same false connections because they don't understand the junk food trap. Once you've understood that junk provides you with no genuine satisfaction, you will start to appreciate the real pleasure of eating your naturally favorite foods and these fears will evaporate. What's more, you'll soon be slim, fit, and healthy, and enjoying life to the full.

Stopping smoking and putting on weight

Ex-smokers who've quit on the willpower method often put on weight as they feel deprived and search for a substitute. If you are one of these people, you may think that you just have to put up with being overweight because you've stopped smoking. This is a myth caused by the brainwashing related to smoking. In fact, nothing could be further from the truth. I was two stone heavier as a smoker. Smoking does not help keep your weight down and with my method you don't have to gain weight when you quit. However, if when you stop smoking, you start substituting with food or alcohol that can lead to a weight problem. If you fall into this category, read my book Stop Smoking Now *as that will remove any lingering feelings of deprivation you may have as a result of quitting smoking and remove the tendency to substitute.*

The favorite foods Nature provides for us can be eaten raw. Even some grains can be soaked and eaten raw. Overcooking destroys the nutritional value of natural foods, so if they are cooked, they should be cooked lightly.

You have been brainwashed into believing that you love foods such as desserts, cakes, and confectionery. But you know they don't love you. Worse than that, they're out to kill you. Do you really want to eat this processed, indigestible, nutritionless, addictive, insulin-triggering junk which clogs up your system, leaves you dissatisfied, and makes you fat?

When we're babies, our bodies produce lactase, the enzyme which can break down lactose making it possible for us to digest the only dairy product we are meant to consume, our mother's milk. We stop producing lactase when we stop feeding from our mother's breast. After infancy we're not designed to consume any dairy products, let alone those of another species. Our body simply can't digest them properly and they turn to fat.

There are foods that genuinely love you and care for you, foods that will look after you throughout your life, keeping you healthy, strong, and slim.

When I was a junk food junkie and very overweight, I hardly ever touched fruit and considered vegetables more as decoration than food. The idea of making them a substantial part of my intake was unimagineable. It was only after I began to understand about Nature's Guide that the prospect became less daunting. Once I realized the extent to which I had been brainwashed, the idea became exciting, and once I started putting my method into practice, the process came naturally and was not only easy but also immensely enjoyable.

All you have to do is open your mind and make the conscious effort to reverse the brainwashing. From now on you will find yourself analyzing processed foods and questioning whether you really want to put them into your body. You'll be amazed at how naturally this comes to you. That's because you're reverting to Nature's plan. What could be more natural than that? You have nothing to fear.

Remember, you can:

Eat as much of your favorite foods as you want, whenever you want, as often as you want, and be the exact weight you want to be without dieting, special exercise, using willpower, or feeling deprived

When you first read this, you were probably very skeptical, perhaps even convinced that it couldn't be true. However, you have read on because you can accept the truth of what I'm saying and you want to see this through. The next step is to make the commitment to do something about it. The eleventh instruction is the most exciting of all:

GO FOR IT!

SUMMARY

• Open your mind and realise you've been brainwashed.

• See junk for what it is.

• See the beauty of your favorite foods.

• Go for it!

Top Tip No.16

Dairy Free

Our digestive system cannot deal with dairy products efficiently. Use oil rather than butter. Use ground nuts and seeds, such as sesame, with a little extra virgin olive oil on your food instead of mayonnaise. Have your tea black or with lemon. Have your coffee black. Or better still, replace your tea and coffee with lemon and water. Eat avocado instead of cheese. It's a natural, high-protein food, full of essential oils.

CHAPTER 17

LAUNCHING YOURSELF

IN THIS CHAPTER
• *WHAT YOU KNOW NOW* • *HUNGER AND ROUTINE*
• *QUENCHING YOUR THIRST*
• *DON'T MIX FOODS THAT FIGHT*

NATURE'S MENU

In the short time it has taken you to read this far, you have learned the principles which will enable you to be slim, fit, and healthy

- You know which foods are in Nature's Guide: fresh fruit, fresh vegetables, fresh seeds, and nuts. They are the easiest for us to digest, can be eaten in their natural state, and have all the nutrients we need. They also taste the best, and can be complemented by whole grains. These are our favorite foods and will keep you slim.

- You know to eat as much raw, high-water-content food as possible.

- You know which foods to beware of: processed foods, especially meat and dairy and those containing processed or refined sugar. Meat and dairy are not suited to the human digestive system and have no nutritional benefits that cannot be obtained much more efficiently from our favorite foods. Processed sugar creates an artificial hunger because of its addictive quality and also clogs up the digestive system. These junk foods give you no genuine pleasure and make you fat.

♦ You know when to eat: when you're hungry. Eating is only a genuine pleasure when you're hungry. Overeating is eating when you're not hungry and gives no satisfaction.

♦ You know when to stop eating: when your hunger is satisfied. You understand the importance of eating slowly, to give your body time to register that it has received the nutrients it needs. You also understand that if you eat junk that doesn't provide the nutrients you need, you will never satisfy your hunger. When you're eating your favorite foods, your Sensor and your Gauge will tell you when you're no longer hungry. Be guided by them.

♦ You know there's no need to set yourself an ideal weight. Wild animals don't and they're never overweight. You'll know when you are the correct weight when you can look in the mirror and be happy with what you see.

♦ You know that dieting doesn't work. By following my method, you will not feel deprived or miserable, and you will be able to enjoy eating.

Any doubts you may have had at the beginning of this book have now been removed. Your mind is open to the most wonderful life change and I'm sure you're itching to get on with it.

Feeling hungry?

Most people eat three meals a day, one in the morning, one around the middle of the day, and one in the evening. This routine is important as it corresponds to the natural cycle of our digestive system, allowing our hunger to build up between meals and so allowing us to enjoy satisfying that hunger when we do eat. It's also convenient for modern living as we can structure our day to enjoy our breakfast, midday, and evening meals with family, friends, or colleagues. Hunger signals start to flow to our brains during the day as the fuel we've consumed at any given meal is used up. If we're eating our favorite foods, we generally become aware of this approximately four or five hours after each meal. Sometimes we may become aware of it between meals and this is no problem since it's a very slight feeling which usually passes very quickly. However, if it persists we can satisfy it by eating a delicious piece of fruit which will quickly be digested and won't ruin our appetite for the meal to come.

It's important to understand that hunger is not to be feared. Hunger is essential to the enjoyment of eating. Satisfying our hunger is a great pleasure and, provided you follow Nature's Guide and my instructions, it's one you can enjoy every day for the rest of your life.

READING NATURE'S GAUGE

Hunger is the gauge Nature has given us to recognize our need for food. So when exactly should we eat?

What if you're not allowed to satisfy your hunger as soon as you sense it? How much of a pain does it become then? Your stomach might rumble I suppose, but that's hardly painful, is it? Any suffering you experience is purely psychological. If you tell yourself you're being deprived, you will feel more miserable and you will regard hunger as a source of misery.

This is why diets are so grueling and ultimately unsuccessful. Because you begin with a sense of deprivation, every time you feel hungry that sense deepens and you feel miserable. That's hardly the right mindset for making a positive change.

I'm not asking you to deprive yourself when you feel hungry. I'm asking you to see hunger in a different light: not as an evil that needs to be dealt with right away but as a source of pleasure that will increase the longer you leave it.

People who pick at food all day tend to believe that it's something in their nature that makes them that way—like a grazing animal. But human beings were not designed to graze. Chimpanzees don't graze, sheep do. We are part of the ape family.

The reason people feel the need to pick at food constantly is because they're permanently hungry—and that's because they're eating the wrong types of food that don't satisfy the body's demand for nutrients.

Start eating the foods that were designed for you and you will find that the desire to keep grazing soon disappears.

Since I'm adamant that we should eat only when we're hungry, does that mean we should do away with the routine of eating three meals a day altogether? Not at all. It's a matter of establishing a routine according to our hunger.

Assuming food is available, wild animals eat whenever they feel like it and don't eat when they don't feel like it. But they still have their own routines that are geared to their needs. Sheep graze all day because that suits their digestive system. Lions tend to eat once a day and then sleep it off. From now on you're going to make the timing, volume, and substance of meals suit your own selfish needs.

THE MOST REFRESHING DRINK IS COOL, CLEAR WATER

If you're really thirsty any drink will be welcome, but the only one that will really quench your thirst is water. Alcohol, nonherbal tea and coffee, fizzy drinks (low-calorie or otherwise), and all processed drinks are mainly water, but they contain additives, drugs, chemicals, and artificial flavorings which do the exact opposite of satisfying your thirst. Big Food markets its drinks as refreshing and rehydrating, but it knows they're making you thirsty. We are the only species on Earth which in adulthood drinks anything other than cool, clear, oxygen-packed water. In Nature's Guide water is the only drink for all animals.

Alcohol is an addictive drug. If you would like to learn how to solve your alcohol problem, you can read *Allen Carr's Easy Way to Control Alcohol*, *Allen Carr's No More Hangovers,* or attend one of our clinics. Coffee and nonherbal tea both contain caffeine which is also an addictive drug. They are also both diuretics, which make you urinate more—lowering their ability to hydrate you. When you drink them, you will crave more and more, not only because they're not quenching your thirst but also because they're addictive. When you take an addictive drug all you are doing is relieving the withdrawal symptoms from the previous dose. You will never be satisfied and you will continue to take it over and over again. When you quench your thirst with water, you're giving your body the nutrients that it's asking for and you will be satisfied. Water is our favorite drink; not only is it refreshing, it's nutritious. Our body is around 60% water and by eating our favorite, high-water-content foods—especially fruit— and drinking water when we're thirsty, we make sure that we do not dehydrate. Water is the lubricant that keeps all our muscles and organs working efficiently and our digestive system relies on liquids to run smoothly.

DON'T MIX FOODS THAT FIGHT

Up until now we've focused on identifying our favorite foods and only eating when we're hungry. If you satisfy your hunger with your favorite foods, then you will solve your problem.

However, there is another factor that needs to be taken into consideration: the correct combination of different types of food. Foods fall into three basic groups: proteins, starches, and neutral foods. If you eat these foods in the right combination, you will improve your digestion, absorption, metabolism, and elimination and, provided you're supplying your body with the right nutrients by eating enough of your favorite foods, you will rebalance your system and reach your ideal body weight.

BETTER DIGESTION

Our bodies use fluids to aid digestion. Different fluids digest different types of food. Protein is digested by acid fluids, whereas starch is digested by alkaline fluids.

Acid is the opposite of alkaline and when the two combine, they counteract each other. If we combine protein and starch in the stomach, both the acid and the alkaline digestive juices are released. These then mix with each other and become ineffective, undermining the efficiency of the digestive process and leading to weight gain.

Proteins should therefore not be eaten with starches. Neutral foods can be efficiently digested with proteins or starches. See the table overleaf.

These guidelines are easy to remember. Follow them and you'll find every meal enjoyable and health-giving. You will also lose weight. With my method there are no feelings of deprivation or misery—only health, energy, and joy!

COLUMN A – PROTEINS	COLUMN B – NEUTRAL	COLUMN C – STARCHES
Meat	Vegetables (except those in C)	Potatoes and Sweet Potatotes
Fish	Seeds	Grains
Shellfish	Nuts	Sweetcorn
Eggs	Herbs	Flour Products
Dairy	Fats and Oils	Bread and Crackers
Soya	Pulses	Pastry

1. Mixing the proteins in column **A** with anything from **column B** is fine.
2. Mixing the starches in column **C** with anything from **column B** is also fine.
3. Mixing the proteins in column **A** with the starches in **column C** causes problems.

Pulses, i.e. dried lentils, beans, peas, and chickpeas, are an exception; they combine well with other vegetables and starches but not with other proteins.

Fruit and fruit juices should not be consumed with any other foods. They should be consumed on an empty stomach and allowed to digest before any other food is eaten. Fruits are digested within 30 minutes, except bananas which can take up to 45 minutes.

SUMMARY

- You now know the principles of my method. Use them!
- Nature gave you a hunger Gauge. Use it!
- Water is a free gift from Nature. Use it!
- You now know the principles of food combining. Use them!
- You now have the knowledge necessary to solve your weight problem. Use it!

Top Tip No.17

Combining

You now have an outline of how to eat. Once you start following these principles it will soon become second nature. You'll find that you don't have to refer to Easyway. You'll enjoy eating a large selection of your favorite foods and mealtimes will be a source of guiltless pleasure. This way of eating is not a diet. Instead of restricting you, it leaves you free to eat your favorite foods.

CHAPTER 18

THE FINAL INSTRUCTION

ENJOY LIFE SLIM

Eating is a source of genuine enjoyment and I want you to enjoy life to the full. You will only be able to do that if you're eating your favorite foods—the foods intended for you by Nature

Unlike diets, which you ultimately give up on as your willpower runs out, my method involves no deprivation and you know you've already solved your weight problem simply by getting it under way.

The Easy Way to Lose Weight solves your weight problem the moment you understand and start following the method.

Your ideal weight is no longer by any means an unattainable goal but a natural and inevitable consequence of your new way of eating.

It's an easy change to make because the foods designed for us by Nature taste the best and you'll find that you quickly recognize them as your favourites.

FRUIT

When you choose to satisfy your hunger is now down to you. The routine of three meals a day is convenient for most people and insures that you allow your hunger to build up so that you enjoy every meal. There's only one rule you should observe concerning timing, and that is to make sure you eat fruit when your stomach does not contain any other food. To get the maximum benefit from fresh fruit it should be digested on its own, so wait at least two hours after eating other foods before consuming fruit. You should also allow at least half an hour for fruit to digest before you eat any other type of food.

Begin your new life by eating fruit, and only fruit, for breakfast. You will find this easy and enjoyable. The conditions are perfect. You won't have eaten since the previous evening. Your stomach will be empty and ready to make the most of the fresh, juicy, delicious, thirst-quenching, nutrient-packed and energy-giving fruit. It will leave you completely satisfied.

Eat your fruit raw. Cooking changes the chemistry of fruit. The heat destroys important enzymes and vitamins, acid is formed, and the nutritional value is lost.

No other breakfast can offer the variety of fruit. You might think you're spoilt for choice in the cereal aisle of your local supermarket, but aren't most of those options just the same thing molded into different shapes, sprinkled with sugar, and all tasting pretty much the same? Head over to the fruit section and look at your options. You'll find at least 20 different fresh fruits, all with their own distinct flavor, all in their natural state, ready to eat, smelling delicious and looking fantastic. You can eat as many as you want and you will not put on weight.

Once you're in the groove of eating only fresh fruit for breakfast, in no time at all it will become second nature and you'll see the combination of egg, bacon, sausage and toast as the mass of greasy, indigestible junk that it really is, and it will have no appeal at all.

I should say first nature, as you know that this is the ideal natural food designed for you and as you rediscover the pleasure of eating that delicious, juicy, nutrient-packed, high-water-content fruit and think about the ease with which you're going to digest it and the benefits you're going to derive from it, you'll soon wonder why you ever ate anything else for breakfast.

While this is happening, you will start to see meat, dairy, confectionery, and other processed foods for the junk they really are. You will think about the effects they would have on your body: the difficulty you would have digesting them; the lack of nutrients which would insure they never satisfy your hunger; the way they would sit rotting inside you for days; the lethargy they would cause; and the fat they would ultimately turn into. And you will rejoice that you no longer have to be a slave to this misery.

As you sense the pleasure and enjoy the benefits of your new, healthy life, you will know that my method is working. And because it's easy and enjoyable, you will know that it will go on working. You will feel more energetic; you will enjoy every meal; your scales will show you that the pounds are falling off; your mirror will show you that the unsightly lumps are disappearing;

your hanging clothes will show you that your figure is trimmer; your stomach will tell you that it's finding life a lot easier now that you're giving it the foods designed for it; and your higher energy levels will confirm that your body is functioning more efficiently. You will also find more and more that your taste buds are drawn to natural, healthy foods, and that a growing number of processed foods now turn you off. The counter-brainwashing begins from day one and your progress is unstoppable.

AM I VEGETARIAN?

"Is this going to turn me into a vegetarian?" That's a question that often comes up and I can understand the concern. Before I discovered this method I always felt vegetarians were a bit weird and the idea of ever becoming one made me feel uneasy, similar to becoming a monk. It was the thought of enforced abstinence and self-deprivation that put me off.

When I was a smoker, I was in awe of nonsmokers. It seemed as if they were somehow a different and superior breed of person looking down on me for my weakness and stupidity. In fact, weakness and stupidity had nothing to with it. I had simply been brainwashed by an ingenious con trick into believing that I couldn't cope with life, let alone enjoy it, without cigarettes. When I finally got rid of the brainwashing and quit smoking for good, I realized that in fact I was no different from the millions of other ex-smokers who had successfully escaped from the nicotine trap. Quitting was a purely selfish decision and I'm delighted to say that life as a nonsmoker is infinitely more enjoyable.

The brainwashing about eating meat must have been deeply ingrained because, even after I understood about its harmful effect and realized that we're not cut out for it, the idea of committing myself to a life without it still made me uncomfortable.

I stopped eating meat because I could no longer convince myself that I enjoyed it and realized I would enjoy life far more without it. It was certainly not for moral reasons. However, when I see an animal nowadays, the idea of killing it, chopping it up into little bits, and eating it seems a bit weird. In fact, the more you learn about meat production, the less you want to eat it. Serious diseases like BSE and CJD have been enough to put a lot of people off beef. A visit to an abattoir, a battery farm, or a meat factory would finish off many more people's appetite for flesh.

If you do become a vegetarian, it will be for the purely selfish reason that you no longer want to eat meat. The great appeal of my method is that there's no deprivation nor any forbidden foods —remember the Junk Margin. Once the brainwashing has been removed and you see meat and other junk for what it really is, you'll instinctively and naturally stop wanting to clog up your body with indigestible, fat-triggering junk and instead become more and more attracted to the foods that are best for you, foods you know will keep you slim, fit, healthy, and happy.

WHAT, NO RECIPES?

Some people pick up this book expecting to find recipes for meals that are guaranteed to help them lose weight. While it may be common practice to include a recipe section in weight loss books,

I don't feel it would be helpful here. Sometimes the authors also give you weekly diet plans to follow. I feel all this is too restrictive.

One of the fundamental principles of Easyway is freedom: freedom to eat what you want, when you want. If you have to follow the recipes and plans in diet books, you'll find yourself feeling deprived.

Your taste buds will give you the confidence to find the recipes you like by your own trial and error. Some of the most satisfying meals I've had are the ones that were completely unplanned. I have listed the vast array of your favorite foods available in the stores, I encourage you to experiment with them all. The twelfth instruction is:

ENJOY LIFE EATING YOUR FAVORITE FOODS

SUMMARY

• You know your weight problem is solved the moment you start following the method.

• Eat as much healthy, high-water-content food as possible.

• You will only become vegetarian if you want to.

• Enjoy losing weight and being free.

Top Tip No. 18

See the Pounds Fall Off

Try on the clothes you've been struggling to fit into or buy yourself something new and rejoice with the sales clerk when you discover you're a size smaller. Weigh yourself once a week and see the difference. Admire the changes in your figure when you look in the mirror.

CHAPTER 19

ENJOYING LIFE TO THE FULL

IN THIS CHAPTER
• *THE* NATURALIZED *CHECKLIST* • *THE RIGHT TIME TO START*
• *EXERCISING FOR PLEASURE* • *THE NATURAL CYCLE*
• *IT'S MARVELOUS* • *THE INSTRUCTIONS*

YOUR PROBLEM SOLVED

The harmonious balance created when you eat the right types of food is a source of health and happiness

You've now received all the information you need to lose weight easily, painlessly, and permanently. So, when do you start?

By now your attitude should be: "Great! My weight problem is solved!"

If you're not yet in that frame of mind, it means you've missed the point somewhere. Review the summaries at the end of each chapter and use our code word, **NATURALIZED,** to help you recap.

NATURALIZED is both a reminder and a checklist. Go through each item and ask yourself, "Do I understand it? Do I agree with it? Do I believe it? Am I following it?" If you have any doubts, reread the relevant chapters.

N	**NEVER** *Feel deprived. You're making no sacrifice.* ***Chapters 1, 6, 7, 11, 16, and 17***
A	**ADVICE** *Ignore it if it conflicts with Nature's Guide.* ***Chapters 4, 6, and 8***
T	**TIMING** *Today!* ***Chapter 19***
U	**UNDERSTAND** *Nature's Guide.* ***Chapters 2, 4, 8, 9, 12, and 16***
R	**REJOICE!** *There's nothing to give up.* ***Chapter 19***
A	**ACCEPT** *that the way you used to eat was making you miserable.* ***Chapter 1***
L	**LIFESTYLE** *Don't change it unless you want to.* ***Chapters 1, and 19***
I	**INTAKE** *your favorite foods.* ***Chapters 1, 6, 7, 12, 14, and 16***
Z	**ZING** *the deliciousness of natural foods.* ***Chapters 7, 14, and 16***
E	**ELEPHANTS** *Don't try not to think about junk.* ***Chapter 19***
D	**DECIDE** *to start now.* ***Chapter 19.***

ALL YOU NEED TO DO IS FOLLOW THE INSTRUCTIONS AND YOU WILL SUCCEED

You have already done all the hard work necessary to reach the right frame of mind. Your preparation is almost complete.

You may now have a feeling of impatience and excitement, like a dog straining at the leash and, if so, that's great. However, you still need to focus carefully on the rest of this book.

Shortly, you'll be taking the decision to change your way of eating for good. When should you do it?

MEANINGLESS DAYS

Two types of occasions often trigger attempts to lose weight. One is a traumatic event such as a health scare or the realization that you've reached a weight or shape that you previously thought unimagineable. The other is a day such as New Year's Day, the start of Lent, or your birthday. I call them meaningless because they have no relation to your weight problem other than to provide a target day to start tackling it. There would be nothing wrong with that if it helped, but meaningless days cause more harm than good.

New Year's Day is by far the most popular meaningless day. We usually eat so much junk around Christmas that we start having trouble doing up our zips. By New Year's Eve we're feeling so bloated and disgusted with ourselves that we're only too pleased to make a resolution. After a few days of carefully controlling our intake, we've recovered from the celebrations and are feeling better. The trouble is that we still hanker after the junk that caused our problems in the first place. If we do manage to lose some weight, the tendency is to "reward" ourselves with more junk. It's like seeing a road accident while we're driving. It may slow us down for few miles, but it's soon put to the back of our mind and we're back up to top speed. Similarly, when we use willpower to go on a diet, we may be determined at first, but as the feeling of deprivation wears us down, we become less and less able to resist going on a binge. There's a constant tug-of-war raging in the overeater's mind. On one side: It's making me fat, lethargic, miserable, unhealthy, and it's controlling my life. On the other side: Boy, do I love eating junk. While the overeater continues to suffer the illusion that junk provides them with a genuine pleasure, they will never escape from this trap.

We're always searching for ways to put off tackling our weight problem because we fear we're going to have to go through some terrible trauma. Meaningless days merely provide us with another excuse to postpone our attempt.

Some people pick a time when they have no social events lined up and hope they won't be tempted. Others choose their annual vacation, thinking that away from the stress of work they'll cope better. The trouble with these approaches is that they leave the lingering doubt: "OK, I've coped so far, but what about that dinner next month?", or "What about when I get back to work?"

NO MATTER WHICH DAY YOU PICK, IT ALWAYS SEEMS TO BE WRONG

With my method you can enjoy meals, drinks, and social occasions right from the start. That way you prove to yourself right away that even during what you feared would be the most difficult times, you're still happy eating your favorite foods and following Nature's Guide.

So, how do you choose the best time to start? Well, what advice would you give your loved ones? It's the same advice they would give you:

"PLEASE START NOW!"

You are fully prepared to start implementing everything you have learned by reading this book. Like the boxer about to win the world title, you are at your peak **NOW**.

If you understand the nature of the trap, there's no reason to delay. So make your decision to start now. If you're hesitating please go through the book again and make sure you understand what each chapter means.

START OFF WITH EXCITEMENT

I realized that if I could put the pleasure back into eating—the genuine, natural pleasure we get from eating our favorite foods —I would find the key to my prison and also help others to escape.

I knew why my method of stopping smoking had become a global success, and so I knew that my method of weight control would also work. Once I realized that the weight problem was caused by eating the wrong foods and consequently overeating and that there was no genuine pleasure in either, I realized that I could successfully apply my method to weight. The key lay in that magical word: pleasure.

On previous attempts to lose weight, my approach had been, "I'm fat and miserable so I'm going to have to eat less, particularly less of the high-calorie, fatty foods which unfortunately I crave most." I was prepared to endure a period of deprivation while I used my willpower to limit my intake, provided I lost weight. And while I stuck at it, the pounds did fall off. But inevitably, eventually my willpower ran out, I reverted to my previous eating habits and the pounds piled back on, resulting in a feeling of frustration and failure and I was even more miserable than before.

This time it was completely different. I realized that if wild animals could eat whatever they wanted, whenever they wanted and be their ideal weight, then I must be able to also. This began the process of opening my mind and getting rid of the brainwashing. When I also realized that the pleasure in eating lay in satisfying my hunger and that junk could never do that, and that, furthermore, there was no pleasure in overeating, I began to see that I would not have to feel deprived. The absence of deprivation meant that I wouldn't have to use willpower, which meant that I had found a permanent solution to my weight problem which involved making no sacrifice. The result was not only to shed the unsightly bulges that I hated, but also to feel fit, healthy, bursting with energy, and, most importantly of all, free from the awful slavery of constantly worrying about my weight.

The objective of this book has been to show you how to do it too. Let's summarize to guarantee your success.

- Animals eat when they're hungry and stop eating when their hunger is satisfied. We've been brainwashed into thinking that there's pleasure in eating purely for eating's sake whether we're hungry or not, and that eating junk gives us genuine pleasure. It's an illusion.

- Use your Gauge and your Sensor to get and stay in touch with your hunger. Hunger is the signal that your body is running low and needs refueling. Hunger gives you the appetite that makes eating enjoyable and food taste delicious. Therefore, hunger is the key to enjoyable eating. Avoid eating when you're not hungry and establish a routine around your hunger. If you find yourself genuinely hungry between meals, have a piece of delicious, fresh fruit.

- You cannot satisfy hunger with junk. Hunger is only satisfied when the body gets the nutrients it needs. If you respond to your hunger by eating junk, you will remain hungry even when you're full. You will not be able to help overeating.

- If there's more on your plate than you have an appetite for, don't eat it. It's not impolite. Monitor your hunger and stop eating when you're satisfied.

- Beware of eating between meals as it will reduce your enjoyment of the next meal. A piece of fruit is fine if you're hungry, but avoid what I call "the peanut trap." This is another social convention that's wrongly regarded as good hosting. There's nothing sociable about laying a trap for your guests that will lure them into overeating. The problem with these foods—I'm talking about salted peanuts, potato chips and similar snacks—is that once you eat one, it's very hard to stop. I would always help myself to a small handful of peanuts, thinking, "I'll just have these and then I'll stop." I would invariably end up finishing the entire bowl. Peanuts in their natural state are very good for you. But the peanuts, potato chips, etc. that are routinely served with drinks are so processed and heavily salted that any lingering nutritional value is far outweighed by the damage they cause.

- Beware of processed foods, in particular processed sugar, which mimics the sweetness of natural fruit, conning us into thinking it's one of our favorite foods when in fact it's an addictive poison.

- Don't try not to think about junk. One of the mistakes we make when we go on a diet is we try not to think about food, with the result that we end up obsessed by it. Trying not to think about something is a fool's game anyway. If I say to you now, "Don't think about elephants," what are you immediately thinking about? Just make sure that whenever you do think about junk, you see it for what it really is.

- Free yourself from the slavery of your current taste buds and the brainwashing of the junk food industry. Be aware that the foods that taste best are those Nature intended for you, the high-water-content foods in their natural state that are best for you, and which will keep you slim, fit, and healthy. These are your favorite foods.

EXERCISING FOR PLEASURE

When I recommend exercise, you may think I've forgotten that I said in Chapter 6 that exercising to lose weight is misguided. I haven't. The more you exercise, the more you need to eat. All animals are designed to take in precisely the amount of fuel they need for the energy they burn off. Furthermore, since muscle is heavier than fat, the net result can actually be weight gain. That's no problem since you won't be setting a target weight and the shift from fat to muscle will transform the unsightly flab into firm, beautiful contours.

However, if you exercise to lose weight, it will have the same psychological effect as going on a diet. It will feel like a hardship.

There's no reason to change your lifestyle unless you want to. I encourage you to exercise, it's healthy for both mind and body, but there are no special exercises needed to achieve your goals and reach your ideal weight.

As you begin to eat more natural foods and your weight drops and your energy level rises, you'll feel a natural urge to be more active. You may develop a greater appetite as a result of doing more. As long as you continue to eat the right foods, this is nothing to worry about because they won't turn into fat but will simply provide the fuel for your more active life. This is the cycle that Nature designed for all creatures, to insure they remain fit, strong, and healthy.

The cycle of healthy eating and activity is not something you have to work at. You will feel it working for you right from the start. Your weight will go down as you're no longer overloading

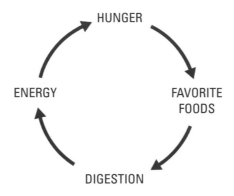

Each phase in the cycle causes the
next. It's the perfect balance—a self-
perpetuating process of pleasure

your body with unwanted junk. You will feel healthier and your
energy levels will rise. It feels great to start the day by stretching
your muscles and getting your circulation going. It creates a
feeling of wellbeing which stays with you all day. Whether you
prefer exercising in the gym or at home, playing sports, or simply
running or walking, it will be enjoyable. Even if you've never
been into sports, as your body becomes lighter, healthier, and
more agile, you'll have more energy and develop a new interest
in exercise. And the more you do it, the more enjoyable it will
become. You don't have to buy machinery, kit yourself out, or pay
to join an expensive gym, you can start by just taking a brisk walk
in the morning. Try to do 20 minutes of exercise a day. In no time
at all you'll be looking forward to the feeling of wellbeing that
exercise brings and before long you'll enjoy the added bonus of
noticing the difference in the mirror.

Don't worry if your appetite increases. Hunger tells us when to eat and a good appetite is a healthy sign and will insure you enjoy your next meal to the full. The food will taste delicious and you'll relish every mouthful. Eating according to Nature's Guide means you will enjoy your food without any guilt whatsoever and will reach and remain your ideal weight.

SOMETHING MARVELOUS IS HAPPENING

The main objective of this book is to show you how to get more pleasure from life, simply by eating the right types of food. I know from my own experience and the countless people who have turned to Easyway for help that nobody is happy being overweight. I believe we were designed to enjoy eating. That's why I did not set out merely with the aim of helping you to lose weight but also proving to you that life will be more enjoyable if you eat your favorite foods.

You'll be slim, healthy, fit, and energetic, and you'll take pride in your reflection in the mirror. As a healthier person, both in mind and body, you'll be better equipped to handle stress and your newly found confidence will transform social occasions.

It's essential for you to realize that you aren't sacrificing anything by following my method and that you are making marvelous positive gains.

My third instruction was: *start off with a feeling of excitement.* Perhaps you found that difficult at the time. You now know there's no reason for doom or gloom. On the contrary, something wonderful is happening. You have every reason to feel excited.

There's no pleasure in self-loathing and lethargy. There's no pleasure in heartburn, indigestion, diarrhoea, and constipation. There's no pleasure in irritable bowels, ulcers, high blood pressure, heart disease, diabetes, and kidney failure. There's no pleasure in being overweight.

Eating junk creates an unbearable tug-of-war. You feel at the same time guilty for eating too much and deprived because you can't eat as much as you want. Fortunately for you, that nightmare is now over. You can now eat as much of your favorite foods as you want and be your ideal weight. Over 99.99% of creatures on this planet do exactly that effortlessly by following Nature's Guide.

Eating natural, healthy food creates a harmonious balance between intake, activity, and appetite. It's a natural cycle and each stage is a pleasure with wonderful benefits. The result of following my method is health and happiness.

Before I discovered a method for solving my weight problem, I felt condemned to a life of pain, sluggishness, guilt, and misery. I had tried dieting, but it only made matters worse. It felt as if I had been imprisoned by my own eating habits and I could see no way out. I even resigned myself to the illusion that, for me and for the millions in my position, it was simply the luck of the draw. Looking back now, I find it difficult to understand how I could have been so blinkered.

The squirrel in my garden made me realize that wild animals know what, when, and how much to eat. They eat their favorite foods, those that Nature designed for them. I realized that every animal on the planet is designed to enjoy eating—you and I included.

As you launch yourself into your new way of life, keep it clear in your mind that you're not making a sacrifice. Eating junk and overeating give you no genuine pleasure or crutch whatsoever. You are not being deprived. It's one of those rare occasions in life when you're making wonderful positive gains and losing nothing at all. There's a huge upside and no downside. Something marvelous is happening to you. So discard any doom or gloom and launch yourself with a feeling of relief that the nightmare is now finally over and excitement at the future. Rejoice that you are now finally free to:

Eat as much of your favorite foods as you want, whenever you want, as often as you want, and be the exact weight you want to be without dieting, special exercise, using willpower, or feeling deprived

SUMMARY

- **Use NATURALIZED to show you the way.**
- **Launch yourself into the method now.**
- **Try exercising. It's an enjoyable part of life.**
- **Enjoy the freedom of eating as Nature intended.**

THE INSTRUCTIONS IN FULL

1 Follow all the instructions.

2 Keep an open mind.

3 Start off with a feeling of excitement.

4 If someone gives you advice that contradicts the advice of Nature, regardless of how eminent or qualified that person may be, IGNORE IT!

5 Don't start off with a preconceived target weight.

6 Do not diet.

7 Only eat when you're hungry.

8 Free yourself from slavery to your current taste buds.

9 Beware of processed foods.

10 Satisfy your hunger with your favorite foods.

11 Go for it!

12 Enjoy life eating your favorite foods.

CHAPTER 20

THE HYPNOTHERAPY

The hypnotherapy CD that comes with this book has been specifically designed to work in conjunction with the book and to help you fully absorb the contents once you have read it. Together they work as a complete and highly effective course that will help you to find it easy to lose weight

Although Allen Carr's Easyway clinics have always used an element of hypnotherapy as part of the process, it's important to stress that it's not the hypnotherapy itself that enables smokers to quit or people to solve their weight problems. The key to the method is removing the illusions brought about by brainwashing. In the case of weight loss, that means removing the illusion that junk food and overeating give you any benefit or pleasure.

Hypnotherapy can be a helpful tool in this process, but it's too simplistic to say that hypnotherapy can stop you from overeating, just as it's too simplistic to say a book can stop you. The key lies in the content of the book and in the content of the hypnotherapy.

A farmer trying to raise crops in an arid part of the world will be thankful for the pipeline that brings water to irrigate his land, but it isn't the pipeline that makes his crops grow, it's the water inside. If the pipeline were carrying oil, it would be useless to the farmer. Hypnotherapy is like a pipeline: It's only effective if its content is right.

You have received the content by reading this book and now

the hypnotherapy is going to help you absorb it. If you haven't yet read the book, please do so before you listen to the CD. It's important that you use the CD and the book together. The hypnotherapy on the CD is completely different from the live experience at Allen Carr's Easyway clinics. It's designed to work as an additional tool to help you absorb the contents of the book, and it will only be effective if you have read the book beforehand.

You may be thinking that you've absorbed all the key messages by reading the book and that you have no need for the CD. Perhaps that's true, but I would still advise you to listen to the hypnotherapy because it will help you to take in all the information you've read in a relaxing and effective way, without any distraction or interruption.

Easyway clinics are specially designed to provide an environment that is geared towards comfort and relaxation. The rooms are furnished with comfortable chairs, lighting is soft, and the temperature is maintained at a pleasant level. Visitors are much more likely to absorb all the information we give them if they're relaxed and not distracted by anything. The mind is much more receptive when it's in this relaxed state. All you have to do is sit back and take it all in.

However, it's not uncommon to be apprehensive about hypnotherapy. People talk about "going under," being "put to sleep," or "losing control." I can reassure you:

NOTHING WEIRD IS GOING TO HAPPEN

You will remain in control throughout the hypnotherapy and there will be no ill effects whatsoever. Some people do drift off to sleep during hypnotherapy, and that's fine because their unconscious mind will still hear and take in the messages. If an emergency were to arise, rest assured that you would respond as normal, even if you have drifted off to sleep. You have absolutely nothing to be concerned about.

The aim, however, is not to go to sleep but just to relax. You may experience a floating feeling or a warm, embracing feeling of deep relaxation, and your thoughts may wander pleasantly as if in a daydream. If so, lucky you. This is a lovely state to be in and highly conducive to absorbing the content of the CD.

If you don't feel yourself drifting off at all, that doesn't mean it's not working. Most people report that nothing much seems to happen, but the hypnotherapy still works for them. All that's required of you is to be nicely relaxed and ready to absorb all the messages that will insure that you solve your weight problem and start enjoying a new life in which food tastes better, you look and feel great, and life is worth celebrating.

THE HYPNOTHERAPY CD WILL NOT BE EFFECTIVE UNLESS YOU HAVE ALREADY READ THE BOOK. IF YOU HAVE NOT ALREADY DONE SO, PLEASE READ THE BOOK BEFORE YOU LISTEN TO THE HYPNOTHERAPY

ALLEN CARR'S EASYWAY CLINICS

The following list indicates the countries where Allen Carr's Easyway To Stop Smoking Clinics are operational at the time of printing.

Check www.allencarr.com for latest additions to this list.

The success rate at the clinics, based on the three-month money-back guarantee, is over 90 percent.

Selected clinics also offer sessions that deal with alcohol, other drugs, and weight issues. Please check with your nearest clinic, listed on the following pages, for details.

Allen Carr's Easyway guarantees that you will find it easy to stop at the clinics or your money back.

JOIN US!

Allen Carr's Easyway Clinics have spread throughout the world with incredible speed and success. Our global network now covers more than 150 cities in over 45 countries. This amazing growth has been achieved entirely organically. Former addicts, just like you, were so impressed by the ease with which they stopped that they felt inspired to contact us to see how they could bring the method to their region.

If you feel the same, contact us for details on how to become an Allen Carr's Easyway To Stop Smoking or an Allen Carr's Easyway To Stop Drinking franchisee.

Email us at: **join-us@allencarr.com** including your full name, postal address, and region of interest.

SUPPORT US!

No, don't send us money!

You have achieved something really wonderful. Every time we hear of someone escaping from the sinking ship, we get a feeling of enormous satisfaction.

It would give us great pleasure to hear that you have freed yourself from the slavery of addiction, so please visit the following web page where you can tell us of your success, inspire others to follow in your footsteps, and hear about ways you can help to spread the word.

www.allencarr.com/444/support-us

You can "like" our Facebook page here: **www.facebook.com/AllenCarr**

Together, we can help further Allen Carr's mission: to cure the world of addiction.

LONDON CLINIC AND WORLDWIDE HEAD OFFICE
Park House, 14 Pepys Road, Raynes Park, London SW20 8NH
Tel: +44 (0)20 8944 7761
Fax: +44 (0)20 8944 8619
Email: mail@allencarr.com
Website: www.allencarr.com
Therapists: John Dicey, Colleen Dwyer, Crispin Hay, Emma Hudson, Rob Fielding, Sam Carroll, Sam Bonner

Worldwide Press Office
Contact: John Dicey
Tel: +44 (0)7970 88 44 52
Email: media@allencarr.com

UK Clinic Information and Central Booking Line
Tel: 0800 389 2115 (UK only)

USA

Central information and bookings:
Toll free: 1 866 666 4299 / New York: 212- 330 9194
Email: info@ theeasywaytostopsmoking.com
Website: www.allencarr.com
Seminars held regularly in New York, Los Angeles, Denver, and Houston
Corporate programs available throughout the U.S.A.
Mailing address: 1133 Broadway, Suite 706, New York, NY 10010
Therapists: Damian O'Hara, Collene Curran, David Skeist

Milwaukee (and South Wisconsin) – opening 2016
Website: www.allencarr.com

New Jersey – opening 2016
Website: www.allencarr.com

CANADA
Toll free: +1-866 666 4299 / +1 905 849 7736
English Therapist: Damian O'Hara

French Therapist: Rejean Belanger
Regular seminars held in Toronto, Vancouver and Montreal
Corporate programs available throughout Canada
Email: info@ theeasywaytostopsmoking.com
Website: www.allencarr.com

UK CLINICS

Belfast
Tel: +44 (0)845 094 3244
Therapist: Tara Evers Choung
Email: tara@easywayni.com
Website: www.allencarr.com

Birmingham
Tel & Fax: +44 (0)121 423 1227
Therapists: John Dicey, Colleen Dwyer, Crispin Hay, Rob Fielding, Sam Carroll
Email: info@allencarr.com
Website: www.allencarr.com

Bournemouth
Tel: 0800 028 7257 (UK only)
Therapists: John Dicey, Colleen Dwyer, Emma Hudson, Sam Carroll
Email: info@allencarr.com
Website: www.allencarr.com

Brighton
Tel: 0800 028 7257 (UK only)
Therapists: John Dicey, Colleen Dwyer, Emma Hudson, Sam Carroll
Email: info@allencarr.com
Website: www.allencarr.com

Bristol
Tel: +44 (0)117 950 1441
Therapist: David Key
Email: stop@easywaysouthwest. com
Website: www.allencarr.com

Cambridge
Tel: +44 (0)20 8944 7761
Therapists: Emma Hudson, Sam Bonner
Email: mail@allencarr.com
Website: www.allencarr.com

Colchester
Tel: +44 (0)1621 819812
Therapist: Lynton Humphries
Email: contact@easywaylynton. com
Website: www.allencarr.com

Coventry
Tel: 0800 321 3007 (UK only)
Therapist: Rob Fielding
Email: info@easywaycoventry. co.uk
Website: www.allencarr.com

Crewe
Tel: +44 (0)1270 664176
Therapist: Debbie Brewer-West
Email: debbie@ easyway2stopsmoking.co.uk
Website: www.allencarr.com

Cumbria
Tel: 0800 077 6187 (UK only)
Therapist: Mark Keen
Email: mark@easywaycumbria. co.uk
Website: www.allencarr.com

Derby
Tel: +44 (0)1270 664176
Therapists: Debbie Brewer-West
Email: debbie@ easyway2stopsmoking.co.uk
Website: www.allencarr.com

Guernsey
Tel: 0800 077 6187 (UK only)
Therapist: Mark Keen
Email: mark@easywaylancashire. co.uk
Website: www.allencarr.com

Ipswich
Tel: +44 (0)1621 819812

Therapist: Lynton Humphries
Email: contact@easywaylynton.
com
Website: www.allencarr.com

Isle of Man
Tel: 0800 077 6187 (UK only)
Therapist: Mark Keen
Email: mark@easywaylancashire.
co.uk
Website: www.allencarr.com

Jersey
Tel: 0800 077 6187 (UK only)
Therapist: Mark Keen
Email: mark@easywaylancashire.
co.uk
Website: www.allencarr.com

Kent
Tel: 0800 028 7257 (UK only)
Therapists: John Dicey, Colleen
Dwyer, Emma Hudson, Sam
Carroll
Email: info@allencarr.com
Website: www.allencarr.com

Lancashire
Tel: 0800 077 6187 (UK only)
Therapist: Mark Keen
Email: mark@easywaylancashire.
co.uk
Website: www.allencarr.com

Leeds
Tel: 0800 077 6187 (UK only)
Therapist: Mark Keen
Email: mark@easywaylancashire.
co.uk
Website: www.ALLENCARR.com

Leicester
Tel: 0800 321 3007 (UK only)
Therapist: Rob Fielding
Email: info@easywayleicester.
co.uk
Website: www.allencarr.com

Lincoln
Tel: 0800 321 3007 (UK only)

Therapist: Rob Fielding
Email: info@easywayleicester.
co.uk
Website: www.allencarr.com

Liverpool
Tel: 0800 077 6187 (UK only)
Therapist: Mark Keen
Email: mark@easywayliverpool.
co.uk
Website: www.allencarr.com

Manchester
Tel: 0800 077 6187 (UK only)
Therapist: Mark Keen
Email: mark@easywaylancashire.
co.uk
Website: www.allencarr.com

**Manchester – alcohol
sessions**
Tel: +44 (0)7936 712942
Therapist: Mike Connolly
Email: info@stopdrinkingnorth.
co.uk
Website: www.allencarr.com

Milton Keynes
Tel: +44 (0)20 8944 7761
Therapists: Emma Hudson, Sam
Bonner
Email: mail@allencarr.com
Website: www.allencarr.com

Newcastle/North East
Tel: 0800 077 6187 (UK only)
Therapist: Mark Keen
Email: info@easywaynortheast.
co.uk
Website: www.allencarr.com

Nottingham
Tel: +44 (0)1270 664176
Therapist: Debbie Brewer-West
Email: debbie@
easyway2stopsmoking.co.uk
Website: www.allencarr.com

Oxford
Tel: +44 (0)20 8944 7761

Therapists: Emma Hudson, Sam
Bonner
Email: mail@allencarr.com
Website: www.allencarr.com

Reading
Tel: 0800 028 7257 (UK only)
Therapists: John Dicey, Colleen
Dwyer, Emma Hudson, Sam
Carroll
Email: info@allencarr.com
Website: www.allencarr.com

**SCOTLAND
Glasgow and Edinburgh**
Tel: +44 (0)131 449 7858
Therapists: Paul Melvin and Jim
McCreadie
Email: info@easywayscotland.
co.uk
Website: www.allencarr.com

Sheffield
Tel: +44 (0)1924 830768
Therapist: Joseph Spencer
Email: joseph@easywaysheffield.
co.uk
Website: www.allencarr.com

Shrewsbury
Tel: +44 (0)1270 664176
Therapist: Debbie Brewer-West
Email: debbie@
easyway2stopsmoking.co.uk
Website: www.allencarr.com

Southampton
Tel: 0800 028 7257 (UK only)
Therapists: John Dicey, Colleen
Dwyer, Emma Hudson, Sam
Carroll
Email: info@allencarr.com
Website: www.allencarr.com

Southport
Tel: 0800 077 6187 (UK only)
Therapist: Mark Keen
Email: mark@easywaylancashire.
co.uk

Website: www.allencarr.com

Staines/Heathrow
Tel: 0800 028 7257 (UK only)
Therapists: John Dicey, Colleen
Dwyer, Emma Hudson, Sam
Carroll
Email: info@allencarr.com
Website: www.allencarr.com

Stevenage
Tel: +44 (0)20 8944 7761
Therapists: Emma Hudson, Sam
Bonner
Email: mail@allencarr.com
Website: www.allencarr.com

Stoke
Tel: +44 (0)1270 664176
Therapist: Debbie Brewer-West
Email: debbie@
easyway2stopsmoking.co.uk
Website: www.allencarr.com

Surrey
Park House, 14 Pepys Road,
Raynes Park, London SW20
8NH
Tel: +44 (0)20 8944 7761
Fax: +44 (0)20 8944 8619
Therapists: John Dicey, Colleen
Dwyer, Crispin Hay, Emma
Hudson, Rob Fielding, Sam
Carroll
Email: mail@allencarr.com
Website: www.allencarr.com

Swindon
Tel: +44 (0)117 950 1441
Therapist: David Key
Email: stopsmoking@
easywaybristol.co.uk
Website: www.allencarr.com

Telford
Tel: +44 (0)1270 664176
Therapist: Debbie Brewer-West
Email: debbie@
easyway2stopsmoking.co.uk
Website: www.allencarr.com

Watford
Tel: +44 (0)20 8944 7761
Therapists: Emma Hudson, Sam
Bonner
Email: mail@allencarr.com
Website: www.allencarr.com

WORLDWIDE CLINICS

REPUBLIC OF IRELAND
Dublin and Cork
Lo-Call (From ROI) 1 890 ESYWAY
(37 99 29)
Tel: +363 (0)1 400 0010 (4 lines)
Therapists: Brenda Sweeney and
Team
Email: info@allencarr.ie
Website: www.allencarr.com

AUSTRALIA
Queensland
Tel: 1300 848 028
Therapist: Natalie Clays
Email: natalie@allencarr.com.auu
Website: www.allencarr.com
Northern Territory – Darwin
Tel: 1300 55 78 01
Therapist: Dianne Fisher and
Natalie Clays
Email: wa@allencarr.com.au
Website: www.allencarr.com

**New South Wales, Sydney,
A.C.T.**
Tel & Fax: 1300 848 028
Therapist: Natalie Clays
Email: natalie@allencarr.com.au
Website: www.allencarr.com

South Australia – Adelaide
Tel: 1300 848 028
Therapist: Jaime Reed
Email: sa@allencarr.au
Website: www.allencarr.com

Victoria
Tel: +61 (0)3 9894 8866 or 1300
790 565
Therapist: Gail Morris

Email: vic@allencarr.com.au
Website: www.allencarr.com

Western Australia – Perth
Tel: 1300 55 78 01
Therapist: Dianne Fisher
Email: wa@allencarr.com.au
Website: www.allencarr.com

AUSTRIA
Sessions held throughout Austria
Freephone: 0800RAUCHEN (0800
7282436)
Tel: +43 (0)3512 44755
Therapists: Erich Kellermann and
Team
Email: info@allen-carr.at
Website: www.allencarr.com

BELGIUM
Antwerp
Tel: +32 (0)3 281 6255
Fax: +32 (0)3 744 0608
Therapist: Dirk Nielandt
Email: info@allencarr.be
Website: www.allencarr.com

BRAZIL
São Paulo
Therapists: Alberto Steinberg &
Lilian Brunstein
Email: contato@easywaysp.
com.br
Tel Lilian - (55) (11) 99456-0153
Tel Alberto - (55) (11) 99325-6514
Website: www.allencarr.com

BULGARIA
Tel: 0800 14104 / +359 899 88
99 07
Therapist: Rumyana Kostadinova
Email: rk@nepushaveche.com
Website: www.allencarr.com

CHILE
Tel: +56 2 4744587
Therapist: Claudia Sarmiento
Email: contacto@allencarr.cl
Website: www.allencarr.com

COLOMBIA – Bogota
Therapist: – Felipe Sanint
  Echeverri
Tel: +57 3158681043
E-mail: info@nomascigarillos.com
Website: www.allencarr.com
CZECH REPUBLIC – opening 2016
  Website: www.allencarr.com

DENMARK
Sessions held throughout
  Denmark
Tel: +45 70267711
Therapist: Mette Fonss
Email: mette@easyway.dk
Website: www.allencarr.com

ECUADOR
Tel & Fax: +593 (0)2 2820 920
Therapist: Ingrid Wittich
Email: toisan@pi.pro.ec
Website: www.allencarr.com

ESTONIA
Tel: +372 733 0044
Therapist: Henry Jakobson
Email: info@allencarr.ee
Website: www.allencarr.com

FINLAND
Tel: +358-(0)45 3544099
Therapist: Janne Ström
Email: info@allencarr.fi
Website: www.allencarr.com

FRANCE
Sessions held throughout France
Freephone: 0800 386387
Tel: +33 (4) 91 33 54 55
Email: info@allencarr.fr
Website: www.allencarr.com

GERMANY
Sessions held throughout
  Germany
Freephone: 08000RAUCHEN
  (0800 07282436)
Tel: +49 (0) 8031 90190-0
Therapists: Erich Kellermann and Team
Email: info@allen-carr.de

Website: www.allencarr.com

GREECE
Sessions held throughout Greece
Tel: +30 210 5224087
Therapist: Panos Tzouras
Email: panos@allencarr.gr
Website: www.allencarr.com

GUATEMALA
Tel: +502 2362 0000
Therapist: Michelle Binford
Email: bienvenid@
  dejedefumarfacil.com
Website: www.allencarr.com

HONG KONG
Email: info@easywayhongkong.
  com
Website: www.allencarr.com

HUNGARY
Seminars in Budapest and 12
  other cities across Hungary
Tel: 06 80 624 426 (freephone) or
  +36 20 580 9244
Therapist: Gabor Szasz and
  Gyorgy Domjan
Email: szasz.gabor@allencarr.hu
Website: www.allencarr.com

ICELAND
Reykjavik
Tel: +354 588 7060
Therapist: Petur Einarsson
Email: easyway@easyway.is
Website: www.allencarr.com

INDIA
Bangalore & Chennai
Tel: +91 (0)80 41603838
Therapist: Suresh Shottam
Email: info@
  easywaytostopsmoking.co.in
Website: www.allencarr.com

ISRAEL
Sessions held throughout Israel
Tel: +972 (0)3 6212525
Therapists: Ramy Romanovsky,
  Orit Rozen, Kinneret Triffon

Email: info@allencarr.co.il
Website: www.allencarr.com

ITALY
Sessions held throughout Italy
Tel/Fax: +39 (0)2 7060 2438
Therapists: Francesca Cesati and
  Team
Email: info@easywayitalia.com
Website: www.allencarr.com

JAPAN
Sessions held throughout Japan
www.allencarr.com

LEBANON
Tel/Fax: +961 1 791 5565
Mob: +961 76 789555
Therapist: Sadek El-Assaad
Email: stopsmoking@allencarr.
  com.lb
Website: www.allencarr.com

LITHUANIA
Tel: +370 694 29591
Therapist: Evaldas Zvirblis
Email: info@mestirukyti.eu
Website: www.allencarr.com

MAURITIUS
Tel: +230 5727 5103
Therapist: Heidi Hoareau
Email: info@allencarr.mu
Website: www.allencarr.com

MEXICO
Sessions held throughout Mexico
Tel: +52 55 2623 0631
Therapists: Jorge Davo and Mario
  Campuzano Otero
Email: info@allencarr-mexico.com
Website: www.allencarr.com

NETHERLANDS
Sessions held throughout the
  Netherlands
Allen Carr's Easyway 'stoppen
  met roken'
Tel: (+31)53 478 43 62 /(+31)900
  786 77 37
Email: info@allencarr.nl

Website: www.allencarr.com

NEW ZEALAND
North Island – Auckland
Tel: +64 (0)9 817 5396
Therapist: Vickie Macrae
Email: vickie@easywaynz.co.nz
Website: www.allencarr.com

South Island – Christchurch
Tel: 0800 327992
Therapist: Laurence Cooke
Email: laurence@
easywaysouthisland.co.nz
Website: www.allencarr.com

NORWAY
Oslo
Tel: +47 93 20 09 11
Therapist: René Adde
Email: post@easyway-norge.no
Website: www.allencarr.com

PERU
Lima
Tel: +511 637 7310
Therapist: Luis Loranca
Email: lloranca@
dejardefumaraltoque.com
Website: www.allencarr.com

POLAND
Sessions held throughout Poland
Tel: +48 (0)22 621 36 11
Therapist: Anna Kabat
Email: info@allen-carr.pl
Website: www.allencarr.com

PORTUGAL
Oporto
Tel: +351 22 9958698
Therapist: Ria Slof
Email: info@comodeixardefumar.
com
Website: www.allencarr.com

ROMANIA
Tel: +40 (0) 7321 3 8383
Therapist: Diana Vasiliu
Email: raspunsuri@allencarr.ro
Website: www.allencarr.com

RUSSIA
Moscow
Tel: +7 495 644 64 26
Therapist: Alexander Formin
Email: info@allencarr.ru
Website: www.allencarr.com
Crimea, Simferopol
Tel: +38 095 781 8180
Therapist: Yuriy Zhvakolyuk
Email: zhvakolyuk@gmail.com
Website: www.allencarr.com
St Petersburg – opening 2016
Website: www.allencarr.com

SERBIA
Belgrade
Tel: +381 (0)11 308 8686
Email: office@allencarr.co.rs
Website: www.allencarr.com

SINGAPORE
Tel: +65 6329 9660
Therapist: Pam Oei
Email: pam@allencarr.com.sg
Website: www.allencarr.com

SLOVAKIA – opening 2016
Website: www.allencarr.com

SLOVENIA
Tel: 00386 (0) 40 77 61 77
Therapist: Gregor Server
Email: easyway@easyway.si
Website: www.allencarr.com

SOUTH AFRICA
Sessions held throughout South
Africa
National Booking Line: 0861
100 200
Head Office: 15 Draper Square, .
Draper St, Claremont 7708,
Cape Town
Cape Town: Dr Charles Nel
Tel: +27 (0)21 851 5883
Mobile: 083 600 5555
Therapists: Dr Charles Nel,
Malcolm Robinson and Team
Email: easyway@allencarr.co.za
Website: www.allencarr.com

SOUTH KOREA
Seoul
Tel: +82 (0)70 4227 1862
Therapist: Yousung Cha
Email: yscha08@gmail.com
Website: www.allencarr.com

SPAIN
Madrid
Tel: +34 91 6296030
Therapist: Lola Camacho
Email: info@dejardefumar.org
Website: www.allencarr.com

SWEDEN
Tel: +46 70 695 6850
Therpaists: Nina Ljungqvist,
Renée Johansson
Email: info@easyway.nu
Website: www.allencarr.com

SWITZERLAND
Sessions held throughout
Switzerland
Freephone: 0800RAUCHEN
(0800/728 2436)
Tel: +41 (0)52 383 3773
Fax: +41 (0)52 3833774
Therapists: Cyrill Argast and
team
For sessions in Suisse Romand
and Svizzera Italiana:
Tel: 0800 386 387
Email: info@allen-carr.ch
Website: www.allencarr.com

TURKEY
Sessions held throughout Turkey
Tel: +90 212 358 5307
Therapist: Emre Ustunucar
Email: info@allencarrturkiye.com
Website: www.allencarr.com

UKRAINE
Kiev
Tel: +38 044 353 2934
Therapist: Kirill Stekhin
Email: kirill@allencarr.kiev.ua
Website: www.allencarr.com

OTHER ALLEN CARR PUBLICATIONS

Allen Carr's revolutionary Easyway method is available in a wide variety of formats, including digitally as audiobooks and ebooks, and has been successfully applied to a broad range of subjects.

For more information about Easyway publications, please visit
www.easywaypublishing.com

The Easy Way for Women to Lose Weight
ISBN: 978-1-78599-458-6 (coming in 2016)

Stop Smoking Now (with hypnotherapy CD)
ISBN: 978-1-78404-542-5

Your Personal Stop Smoking Plan
ISBN: 978-1-78404-833-4

Stop Smoking with Allen Carr (with 70-minute audio CD)
ISBN: 978-1-78599-146-2

The Easy Way for Women to Stop Smoking
ISBN: 978-1-84837-464-5

Stop Drinking Now
ISBN: 978-1-78404-541-8

The Easy Way for Women to Stop Drinking
ISBN: 978-1-78599-147-9

The Easy Way to Stop Gambling
ISBN: 978-1-78212-448-1

The Easy Way to Control Alcohol
ISBN: 978-1-84837-465-2

Good Sugar Bad Sugar
ISBN: 978-1-78599-459-3 (coming in 2016)

Allen Carr's Get Out of Debt Now
ISBN: 978-1-84837-981-7

The Easy Way to Enjoy Flying
ISBN: 978-0-71819-458-3

How to Stop Your Child Smoking
ISBN: 978-0-14027-836-1

The Easy Way to Stop Smoking
ISBN: 978-0-71819-455-0

The Only Way to Stop Smoking Permanently
ISBN: 978-0-14-024475-1

Packing It In The Easy Way (the autobiography)
ISBN: 978-0-14101-517-0

Finally Free!
ISBN: 978-1-84858-979-7

The Illustrated Easy Way to Stop Smoking
ISBN: 978-1-84837-930-5

The Illustrated Easy Way to Stop Drinking
ISBN: 978-1-78404-504-3

The Illustrated Easy Way for Women to Stop Smoking
ISBN: 978-1-78212-495-5

No More Ashtrays
ISBN: 978-1-84858-083-1

No More Hangovers
ISBN: 978-1-84837-555-0

No More Worrying
ISBN: 978-1-84837-826-1

No More Gambling
ISBN: ebook

No More Debt
ISBN: ebook

No More Fear of Flying
ISBN: 978-1-78404-279-0

No More Diets
ISBN: 978-1-84837-554-3

The Nicotine Conspiracy
ISBN: ebook

Burning Ambition
ISBN: 978-0-14103-030-2

How to Be a Happy Non-Smoker
ISBN: ebook

Smoking Sucks (Parent Guide with 16 page pull-out comic)
ISBN: 978-0-572-03320-0

The Little Book of Quitting
ISBN: 978-1-45490-242-3

Want Easyway on your smartphone or tablet?
Search for "Allen Carr" in your app store.

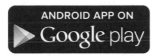 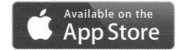

Easyway publications are also available as audiobooks.
Visit www.easywaypublishing.com to find out more.

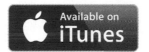 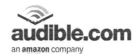

DISCOUNT VOUCHER
for
ALLEN CARR'S
EASYWAY CLINICS

Recover the price of this book when you attend an
Allen Carr's Easyway Clinic
anywhere in the world!

Allen Carr's Easyway has a global network of stop
smoking clinics where we guarantee you'll find it easy
to stop smoking or your money back.

**The success rate based on this
unique money-back guarantee is over 90%.**

Sessions addressing weight, alcohol and other
drug addictions are also available at certain clinics.

When you book your session, mention this
voucher and you'll receive a discount of
the price of this book. Contact your nearest
clinic for more information on how the sessions
work and to book your appointment.

**Details of Allen Carr's Easyway
Clinics can be found at**
www.allencarr.com
or call 1866 666 4299

This offer is not valid in conjunction with any other offer/promotion.